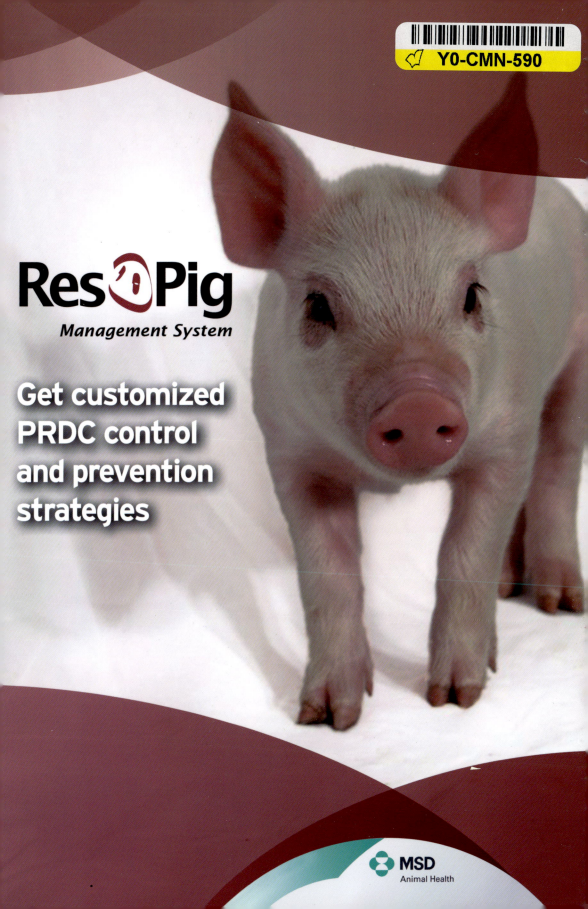

Res Pig
Management System

Get customized PRDC control and prevention strategies

MSD
Animal Health

Make ResPig® your porcine respiratory disease complex (PRDC) decision-making tool

The ResPig® Management System is a web-based platform that identifies areas of improvement, cost and potential outcomes of PRDC control and prevention strategies specific to a farm's needs. Tools include:

- **Farm Audits:** Includes management, health and disease assessments specific to a herd.

- **Slaughter Check Analysis:** Presents a more detailed look at pathogens and disease severity.

- **Economic Simulation:** Provides return on investment (ROI) based on decisions and farm performance.

  - ResPig provides concise reports, conclusions and action items.

  - The herd veterinarian can make additional comments, establish timelines and set targets.

  - The reports can be used to discuss the data and strategies with the producer, and determine how to move forward.

- **Information Resources:** Access to detailed information on PRDC and the associated disease pathogens, including information about MSD Animal Health respiratory vaccines and pharmaceuticals.

Created for you

ResPig was created for veterinarians, farmers and other swine specialists. Extensive updates have made it even more user-friendly, flexible and solutions-oriented. Access can be personalized by country – including language, financials and products. Plus it's now iPad compatible; you can work offline.

MSD Animal Health is committed to PRDC prevention and control by providing effective vaccines, pharmaceuticals, technical support and diagnostic tools, all of which are grouped under the ResPig Management System.

One PRDC solution, many options you can model and evaluate before implementing

There's nothing else quite like ResPig. ResPig gives you comprehensive analysis and solutions. The ResPig web-based platform lets you:

- Model and review options to enhance PRDC prevention and control

- Audit your on-farm management and animal health processes

- Evaluate possible interventions and their ROI

- Receive customized, farm-level recommendations and action plans

- Use the reports to develop targets and monitor progress

Contact your MSD Animal Health representative today to gain PRDC control and prevention strategies, and tools you can use to improve your clients' bottom line.

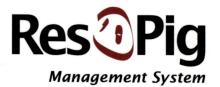

Handbook of laboratory diagnosis in swine

© 2013 Grupo Asís Biomedia S.L.
Plaza Antonio Beltrán Martínez, nº 1, planta 8 - letra I
(Centro empresarial El Trovador)
50002 Zaragoza - Spain

Design and layout:
Servet editorial - Grupo Asís Biomedia, S.L.
www.grupoasis.com
info@grupoasis.com

Printing: Gráficas Lizarra S.L.
ULZAMA gráficas
Pol. Ind. Areta, calle A-35
31620 Huarte, Navarra

D.L.: Z 558-2013

Printed in Spain

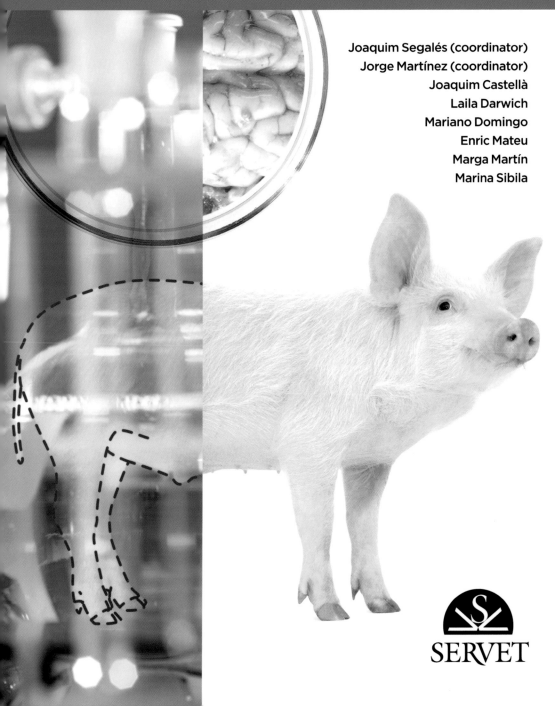

Handbook of laboratory diagnosis in swine

Joaquim Segalés (coordinator)
Jorge Martínez (coordinator)
Joaquim Castellà
Laila Darwich
Mariano Domingo
Enric Mateu
Marga Martín
Marina Sibila

SERVET

Authors

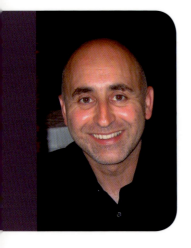

Dr. Joaquim Segalés
DVM, PhD, Dipl. ECVP, Dipl. ECPHM

Dr. Joaquim Segalés was born in Vic (Barcelona), Spain. He obtained his DVM from the *Universitat Autònoma de Barcelona* (UAB) in 1991. In 1996, he was awarded a PhD from the same university. He also conducted his PhD research at the University of Minnesota for 15 months. In 2000 he was board certified by the European College of Veterinary Pathologists (ECVP), and is a founding member of the European College of Porcine Health and Management. Since 1996 he has been working as a professor of Swine Pathology and Clinical Medicine at the UAB. From 1996 to 2012 he was responsible for swine disease diagnosis at the Department of Animal Health and Anatomy of the UAB. In 2000 he joined the *Centre de Recerca en Sanitat Animal* (CReSA, Animal Health Research Centre) as a researcher and has been the director of the centre since 2012.

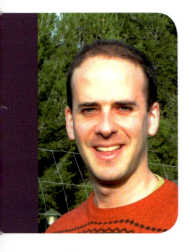

Dr. Jorge Martínez
DVM, PhD, Dipl. ECVP

Dr. Jorge Martínez was born in Valencia, Spain. He obtained his DVM from the *Universidad Cardenal Herrera - CEU*, Valencia, in 2001. In 2006, he was awarded a PhD from the same university for his work on swine health monitoring at slaughter. In 2005, he started his residency in anatomic pathology at the *Universitat Autònoma de Barcelona* (UAB) and in 2010 he was board certified by the European College of Veterinary Pathologists (ECVP). Since 2010 he has been working as a lecturer at the UAB. Most of his research has been focused on swine pathology, particularly respiratory diseases.

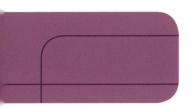

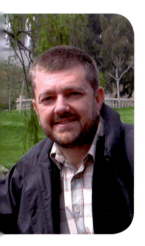

Dr. Joaquim Castellà
DVM, PhD

Dr. Joaquim Castellà was born in Roquetes (Tarragona), Spain. He obtained his DVM from the University of Zaragoza, Spain, in 1987. In 1992, he was awarded a PhD from the *Universitat Autònoma de Barcelona*. He has been working as a lecturer at the Veterinary Faculty of the same university since 1994. Most of his research has focused on veterinary parasitology, particularly veterinary entomology and vector-borne diseases.

Dr. Laila Darwich
DVM, MSc, PhD

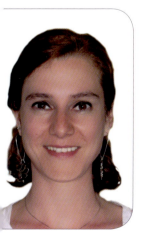

Dr. Laila Darwich was born in Barcelona, Spain. She obtained her DVM (with an award for Excellence in Academic Performance) by the *Universitat Autònoma de Barcelona* (UAB) (1994-1999). In 2001, she completed a master's degree in Veterinary Medicine (UAB) and was awarded a PhD in Veterinary Medicine in 2004. She joined the Juan de la Cierva Programme (2005-2007) with a postdoctoral position at the HIV Clinical Unit, Irsicaixa Foundation (Institute of AIDS Research, *Hospital Germans Trias i Pujol, Badalona*). She has worked as Assistant Professor (2003-2005), Lecturer (2007-2012) and Associate Professor (currently) at the Infectious Disease and Epidemiology Unit (Animal Health Department, Faculty of Veterinary Medicine, UAB) and is a researcher at the *Centre de Recerca en Sanitat Animal* (CReSA, Research Centre in Animal Health). Areas of Expertise: viral immunity and immunopathology of swine and human viruses and epidemiology of infectious diseases.

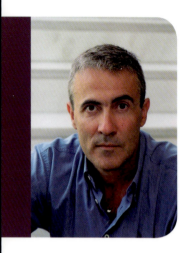

Dr. Mariano Domingo
DVM, PhD, Dipl. ECVP

Dr. Mariano Domingo was born in Madrid, Spain. He obtained his DVM from the University of Zaragoza in 1979. In 1982 he was awarded a PhD by the Justus-Liebig University Giessen, Germany. In 1984 he started teaching and researching in animal pathology at the Veterinary School (*Universitat Autònoma de Barcelona*). In 1995 he became a *de facto* member of the European College of Veterinary Pathologists (ECVP). Most of his research has focused on pathology in different species and more particularly on pig diseases.

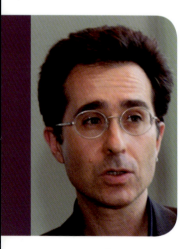

Dr. Enric Mateu
DVM, PhD, Dipl. ECPHM

Dr. Enric Mateu is Professor of Infectious Diseases at the Faculty of Veterinary Medicine of the *Universitat Autònoma de Barcelona* (UAB) and a researcher at the *Centre de Recerca en Sanitat Animal* (CReSA, Animal Health Research Centre) in Barcelona. He earned his degree in Veterinary Medicine in 1989 and was awarded a PhD from the UAB in 1993. He is a diplomate of the European College of Porcine Health and Management. He was a research scholar at the University of Illinois (USA) in 1994-95. His research focuses on swine medicine, particularly viral diseases of swine. He has participated in several projects dealing with porcine circovirus, swine influenza and PRRS and is the author of several international peer-reviewed papers on swine diseases. He is currently participating in the European consortium PoRRSCon (an EU funded project for the development of new tools against PRRS) and the European network EuroPRRSNet.

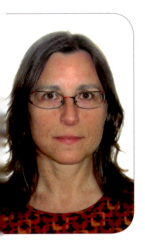

Dr. Marga Martín
DVM, PhD, Dipl. ECPHM

Dr. Marga Martín was born in Barcelona, Spain. She obtained her DVM from the University of Zaragoza (Spain) in 1984. In 1992 she was awarded a PhD from the *Universitat Autònoma de Barcelona* (UAB) for her work on the epidemiology of coronavirus infections in pigs. Since 1993 she has worked as Professor of Animal Health at the Faculty of Veterinary Medicine of the UAB, teaching mainly about infectious diseases in pigs, poultry and carnivores. In 2009 she was board certified by the European College of Porcine Health Management (ECPHM). Most of her research has focused on viral and bacterial infections in pigs.

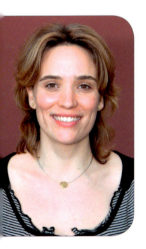

Dr. Marina Sibila
Biologist, PhD, DVM

Dr. Marina Sibila, a researcher at the CReSA since 2004, has an extensive background in molecular epidemiology of swine respiratory pathogens. Her PhD research, carried out at the Faculty of Veterinary Medicine of the *Universitat Autònoma de Barcelona*, focused on the molecular epidemiology of *Mycoplasma hyopneumoniae* infections under field conditions. In the past few years, she has gained broad experience in other economically important swine respiratory pathogens such as *Actinobacillus pleuropneumoniae*, *Haemophilus parasuis* and porcine circovirus type 2 (PCV2) under field and experimental conditions. She has been involved in the publication of more than 39 peer-reviewed papers (49% of them on PCV2 research).

Preface

Laboratory analyses are of great help to make a definitive diagnosis of a disease or poor production problem. A correct and precise diagnosis allows the establishment of preventive and control measures (management, breeding, animal flow, therapies, vaccination schedules, etc.) with a high probability of success. Therefore, a global diagnostic approach is perceived, both by the veterinary clinician and farmer, as a paramount action when dealing with diseases. The cost of the diagnostic effort is minimal, taking into account the losses caused by an overt disease or sub-optimal production that remains incorrectly diagnosed. As a consequence, the establishment of a precise diagnosis is always useful from a return on investment point of view. It is important to note that the accuracy of the diagnosis depends on the correct interpretation of the obtained data, regardless of whether these come from clinical observations, epidemiological assessment, pathological findings or laboratory analyses.

Assuming that veterinary clinicians are usually well trained in terms of clinical, epidemiological and pathological data analysis, the main aim of the present guide is to provide a broad view of all the aspects of laboratory analysis to diagnose swine diseases. Analyses are not just "kitchen work" in a laboratory, and the results obtained are not only the consequence of a "well-performed technique". Veterinary clinicians need to understand that diagnostic laboratories will be able to help them as long as samples are properly selected, collected and submitted. Moreover, laboratories cannot test everything and the submitting vet should know what can and cannot be done from an analytical point of view in the chosen laboratory. This requires close collaboration between veterinary surgeons and laboratory personnel. Veterinary clinicians should know how to interpret the results of the analyses, and we truly believe that this can only be achieved with a comprehensive knowledge of what each technique offers.

To summarise, this guide is aimed at helping both veterinary clinicians and students. As personnel involved in diagnostic laboratory work, we are aware of the extensive knowledge that is necessary when working in the field of swine health and production. Therefore, the present guide offers you updated and practical information on laboratory diagnostic techniques and their usefulness. If you improve your diagnostic skills by reading this handbook, our objective will have been achieved!

The authors
Bellaterra (Barcelona, Spain)
February 2013

Prologue

As a professor, researcher and diagnostician, I have always believed that sharing knowledge, "know-how" and scientific techniques is one of the most important keys to excellence in veterinary medicine. Despite traditional surveillance and prevention techniques, such as serology, slaughterhouse controls and vaccination, some infections and diseases remain at uncontrollable levels and are frequently associated with environmental and management factors. In addition, many diseases have a poorly understood and, most often, complex (multifactorial) cause. The intensification of swine production has also led to subclinical or chronic diseases that usually lead to poor performance rather than clinical disease. Nevertheless, we all know that failure in controlling diseases in a specific herd may also be the consequence of a simply inadequate diagnosis. In other words, science has provided veterinary surgeons with a broad variety of new knowledge during the last few years which, in turn, has complicated their lives when a clear and complete diagnosis must be achieved!

Since production systems are in constant evolution and new diseases are emerging (whereas others are declining), clear updates on the fundamental diagnostic principles are needed. It should be kept in mind that a complete diagnosis may also include detection of non-apparent (sub-clinical) infections that contribute to the knowledge of the spreading of a disease in a specific country or geographical area. In this book, the authors have developed a collection of accessible chapters detailing current knowledge on diagnostic techniques from a practical point of view while retaining the big picture. From clinical examination and sample collection (which many times represents the "Achilles' heel" of a successful laboratory diagnosis), to the differential diagnosis of infectious and non-infectious diseases, this book provides the reader with a simple yet complete and easy-to-read source of applied information on the diagnosis of the most important swine diseases. Complete tables, explanations of pathological terms and highly explicit charts leading to the differential diagnosis of syndromes presenting similar clinical characteristics, are present in each chapter. Targeted readers are mainly veterinary surgeons, but also technicians working in animal disease. The authors of this book are renowned scientists and diagnosticians from the *Centre de Recerca en Sanitat Animal* (CReSA) and Autonomous University of Barcelona (UAB), Spain, with a wide experience in diagnosis of swine diseases. This book should always be available at the veterinary surgeon's fingertips to help them carry out the most accurate diagnosis possible.

Marcelo Gottschalk
Professor, Faculty of Veterinary Medicine
University of Montreal, Québec, Canada

Table of contents

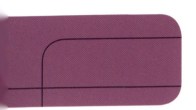

ABBREVIATIONS

ADV: Aujeszky's disease virus/pseudorabies virus.
A. pleuropneumoniae: *Actinobacillus pleuropneumoniae.*
A. pyogenes: *Arcanobacterium pyogenes.*
ASF: African swine fever.
ASFV: African swine fever virus.
A. suis: *Actinobacillus suis.*
A. suum: *Ascaris suum.*
B. bronchiseptica: *Bordetella bronchiseptica.*
B. coli: *Balantidium coli.*
B. hyodysenteriae: *Brachyspira hyodysenteriae.*
B. pilosicoli: *Brachyspira pilosicoli.*
B. suis: *Brucella suis.*
cELISA: competitive enzyme-linked immunosorbent assay.
CK: creatine kinase.
CNS: central nervous system.
CPE: cytopathic effect.
C. perfringens: *Clostridium perfringens.*
CSF: classical swine fever.
CSFV: classical swine fever virus.
E. coli: *Escherichia coli.*
ELISA: enzyme-linked immunosorbent assay.
EMCV: encephalomyocarditis virus.
E. rhusiopathiae: *Erysipelothrix rhusiopathiae.*
FMDV: foot-and-mouth disease virus.
FOD: fibrous osteodystrophy.
HAI: haemagglutination inhibition.
HBS: haemorraghic bowel syndrome.
H. parasuis: *Haemophilus parasuis.*
H. suis: *Haematopinus suis.*
H. rubidus: *Hyostrongylus rubidus.*
IF: immunofluorescence test.
IgA: immunoglobulin A.
IgG: immunoglobulin G.
IgM: immunoglobulin M.
IHC: immunohistochemistry.
IPMA: indirect peroxidase monolayer assay.
ISH: *in situ* hybridisation.
I. suis: *Isospora suis.*
L. biflexa: *Leptospira biflexa.*

L. intracellularis: *Lawsonia intracellularis.*
EM: electron microscopy.
M. flocculare: *Mycoplasma flocculare.*
M. hyopneumoniae: *Mycoplasma hyopneumoniae.*
M. hyorhinis: *Mycoplasma hyorhinis.*
M. hyosinoviae: *Mycoplasma hyosinoviae.*
M. suis: *Mycoplasma (Eperythrozoon) suis.*
MIC: minimum inhibitory concentration.
nPCR: nested PCR.
PAR: progressive atrophic rhinitis.
PCR: polymerase chain reaction.
PCV2: porcine circovirus type 2.
PCV2-SD: PCV2 systemic disease (also known as postweaning multisystemic wasting syndrome).
PDNS: porcine dermatitis and nephropathy syndrome.
PEDV: porcine epidemic diarrhoea virus.
PFTS: peri-weaning failure-to-thrive syndrome.
P. multocida: *Pasteurella multocida.*
PPV: porcine parvovirus.
PRCV: porcine respiratory coronavirus.
PRDC: porcine respiratory disease complex.
PRRS: porcine reproductive and respiratory syndrome.
PRRSV: porcine reproductive and respiratory syndrome virus.
PRV: pseudorabies virus/Aujeszky's disease virus.
qPCR: quantitative or real-time PCR.
RAR: regressive atrophic rhinitis.
RT-PCR: reverse transcription PCR.
SIV: swine influenza virus.
S. choleraesuis: *Salmonella choleraesuis.*
S. hyicus: *Staphylococcus hyicus.*
S. ransomi: *Strongyloides ransomi.*
S. scabiei: *Sarcoptes scabiei.*
S. suis: *Streptococcus suis.*
TGEV: transmissible gastroenteritis virus.
T. gondii: *Toxoplasma gondii.*
T. suis: *Trichuris suis.*
Y. enterocolitica: *Yersinia enterocolitica.*

1

Introduction

INTRODUCTION

In the last 20 years, swine production has become highly specialised, with large, intensive and confinement-rearing production systems. This scenario has been coupled with farmers with a high level of professionalism and education, who demand an outstanding service from their veterinary surgeons and consultants. In parallel, during the same period, pathological problems have evolved to complex disease scenarios, in which old and new pathogens are mixed and interact with management and environmental factors and the production system. Moreover, farmers and veterinary surgeons are not only committed to producing healthy and nutritive food, but also to doing it under animal welfare conditions. It is therefore worth highlighting that production of safe pork products contributing to public health is mainly achievable in a scenario of no or minimal pig disease.

It is true, however, that intensive production systems imply very large concentrations of animals in limited spaces, and the likelihood of being hit by infectious diseases is a permanent threat. Moreover, non-infectious diseases or pathological conditions, such as nutritional deficiencies or toxicities, as well as management problems (water flow, automatic feeding systems, etc.) may also affect a pig population. Overall, a scenario of a complex disease indicates that both farmers and vets must be prepared to face multifactorial disease problems, and a correct and timely diagnosis is the first step to ensure their proper control.

The diagnostic process is a rather complex plan that includes several steps ending with tailor-made prevention or control strategies for a specific pig farm. Within this process, clinical investigation is the cornerstone. A presumptive diagnosis is established by means of clinical and epidemiological data collection. Clinical investigation has two main phases. The first one is the inductive (descriptive) step, and involves answering the questions of "Who has what, where, when, since when, how many and how?". The second one is the deductive step, in which hypotheses on the causality of the problem have to be established. No matter what control or prevention strategy is implemented, it should be the natural and logical consequence of the clinical investigations. In this context, it is important to emphasise that "for each mistake we make by not knowing, we will make ten mistakes by not looking" (Steve Henry, at the annual Meeting of the American Association of Swine Veterinarians, 2003). Therefore, the clinical investigation is key since the entire further diagnostic effort depends on the quality of it.

Clinical investigations might not be enough to have a complete or sufficient picture of what is going on on a farm. Moreover, it might not be sufficient to establish the most efficient and economically feasible strategies to minimise or eliminate the problem. In these cases, further diagnostic investigations are recommended and laboratory analyses may allow the confirmation or ruling out of the contribution of specific infectious agents or toxins. In fact, laboratory testing is mainly used to:

- Detect pathogens or toxins potentially involved in a disease or suboptimal production.
- Evaluate the infection/exposure status of pig individuals or populations.
- Estimate the percentage of herds or pigs with antibodies to a pathogen.
- Monitor a herd serological response to vaccination.
- Monitor the progress and success of disease control or eradication programmes.

The path to get a laboratory result potentially useful for diagnostic and control/prevention purposes is not exempt of complexities. First of all, the veterinary surgeon must make an appropriate selection of animals and samples to be submitted for laboratory investigations. Some clinical samples such as blood, serum and saliva samples, nasal swabs or broncho-alveolar lavages might be collected from live animals, while some others must be taken during the necropsy of pigs that are representative of the disease problem. Important clinical considerations such as the suspected duration of the illness, the treatment history, the availability of animals with the problem and the best time to select animals for testing will be crucial to ensure the most reliable results coming from the laboratory. Chapter 2 of this guide reviews the most important aspects associated with sampling.

Secondly, effective sample collection and submission to the laboratory are also compulsory steps to increase the likelihood of a correct diagnosis. This is an excellent example of how the veterinary surgeon contributes to the reliability of laboratory tests, by providing the right sample in the best condition. Sample submission will be discussed in chapter 3.

Thirdly, the veterinary surgeon must be aware of the existing laboratory tests and their corresponding interpretation. Not all diagnostic laboratories can test everything, so it is very important to establish sound decisions as regards the approach to the analytical plan. The veterinary surgeon must decide on the agents/toxins to be tested (confirmed/ruled out) -by means of his/her presumptive diagnosis- as well as which laboratory to work with, taking into account the availability of tests for each agent in the chosen laboratory, their cost and the time required to get the results back. In any case, veterinary surgeons should call the laboratory for advice before sampling and sample submission. Chapter 4 of this guide summarises the knowledge on the basic laboratory tests, their usefulness and overall interpretation.

Finally, chapters 5 to 10 offer a practical overview of the differential diagnosis of diseases according to body systems in swine. This book does not intend to substitute existing general textbooks on swine diseases or laboratory testing. The ultimate objective of the present guide is to summarise and integrate in a comprehensive manner the different steps necessary to reach a final diagnosis of swine diseases that require laboratory intervention.

2

Sample collection

SAMPLING AT NECROPSY

Several protocols to perform a necropsy in pigs are available. The veterinary surgeon may choose any of these protocols, but it is recommended to follow the same procedure to perform a systematic, complete and organised necropsy. This chapter reviews the methods and types of samples that can be used during the necropsy.

A properly performed necropsy can yield much valuable information about a disease. Gross pathology alone will provide a diagnosis in some cases, but additional testing is often required to obtain a definitive diagnosis. The range of techniques in use is expanding, but traditional methods are still the first line of investigation. Table 1 gives a list of potential samples to be collected at necropsy.

Selection of animals

The best way to ensure an accurate diagnosis is to have fresh and well-preserved samples. It is therefore advised to perform necropsies on recently slaughtered animals, and 3-4 pigs may thus be selected from the population of affected animals. When possible, select those animals in the acute phase of the disease (first 24-48 hours) that represent a pattern of clinical signs that is similar to that of the other members of the group. To avoid any interference with further laboratory analyses, avoid those that have already been treated (at least systemically).

There are several approved protocols to perform ethic euthanasia in pigs; however, intravenous barbiturates are recommended because their price is low and they allow organ preservation.

Blood sampling

Blood samples should be collected *in vivo* (figs. 1 and 2) or just after euthanasia, when the heart is still beating. If several hours have passed after death, heart blood clots may be collected and used for microbiological, virological, PCR or serological analyses.

Different *in vivo* techniques using various sites have been described: anterior vena cava (younger animals, from birth to 2 months of age approximately), jugular vein (fatteners and finishers) and tail or ear veins (adults). Blood samples for haematology and biochemistry should be collected into tubes containing sodium EDTA or lithium heparin. Blood collected into tubes without any anticoagulants is also suitable for most serological and biochemical tests (fig. 3).

Histopathology

Tissue samples for histopathological examination, IHC analysis and ISH should be immersed in 10% neutral buffered formalin and stored at room temperature. The tissue:formalin volume ratio should be no less than 1:10. The sample jars must be clearly labelled with the animal's identification. All the samples from the same animal can be included in the same jar. Use as many jars as the number of necropsied pigs. Tissue samples should be no thicker than 0.5 cm; otherwise the lack of penetration of formalin may favour autolysis (fig. 4). The exception is the brain and eye globe, which are fixed intact. As for the intestine, it is recommended to collect several portions and the samples should be opened longitudinally before being immersed in formalin.

The samples should be taken from the border of the lesions or, alternatively, include affected and non-affected areas of the same organ.

Microbiology/virology/ molecular techniques

Specimens of blood, urine, saliva, milk, cerebrospinal fluid or tissues should be collected as aseptically as possible for culture, virological analysis or PCR tests (figs. 5 and 6).

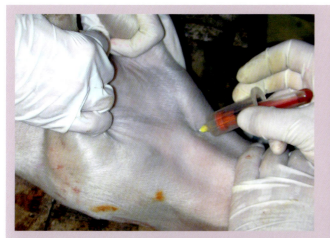

Figure 1. Blood collection *in vivo* from the cranial cava vein.

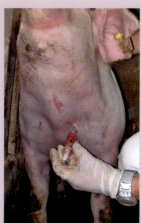

Figure 2. Blood collection *in vivo* from the jugular vein.

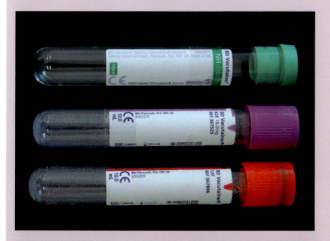

Figure 3. Blood collection tubes for haematology and biochemistry with an anticoagulant (EDTA - pink, heparin - green). Tubes without any anticoagulants (red) are used to obtain serum in order to perform serological or biochemistry tests.

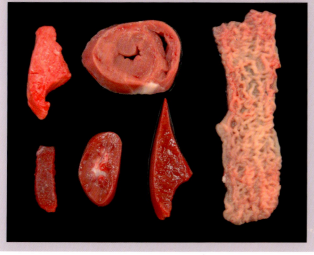

Figure 4. Tissue collection for histopathology. Samples should not be thicker than 0.5 cm to facilitate fixation; the intestine must be longitudinally opened.

In tissue samples, it is recommended to submit a large portion of the organ, since large pieces of tissue allow the laboratory to take aseptic samples. This is the case of the lungs, liver, heart, kidney or spleen. In other cases, when necrosis or exudates are observed, swabs can be taken from these lesions. In cases of meningitis, swabs from the meninges or third ventricle can be collected (fig. 7); submission of the entire brain is also recommended. For the small and large intestines, unopened segments of the gut with their ends tied off should be sent to the laboratory (fig. 8).

Each sample must be kept in separate bags/jars to avoid contamination (fig. 9).

When considering the possible causes of a disease, it is convenient to consult bacteriologists or virologists about how to conserve or submit samples under appropriate conditions: media, temperatures, etc. (chapter 3).

Toxicology

Since there is a huge range of toxic compounds, samples for toxicological analysis must include tissues (liver, kidney and brain), blood, serum, stomach contents or urine from dead animals. In other cases, food or water can be also tested for evidence of toxins. Tissue, serum, urine, stomach contents, food or water may be either refrigerated or frozen, while blood should not be frozen.

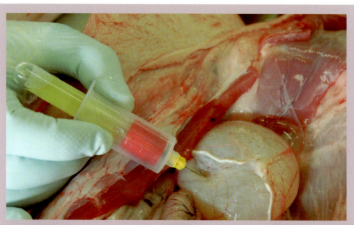

Figure 5. Sterile collection of urine in into tubes with no anticoagulants.

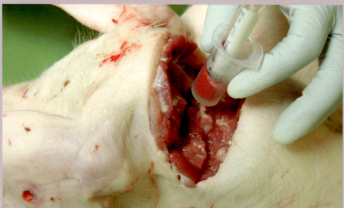

Figure 6. Sterile collection of cerebrospinal fluid from the cisterna magna in the atlanto-occipital joint. The fluid must be transparent, and contamination with blood should be avoided.

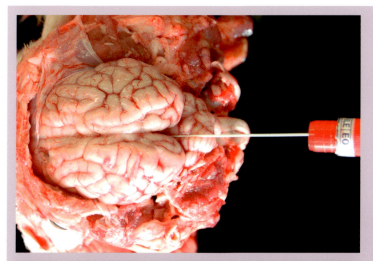

Figure 7. In the case of a suspicion of meningitis, third ventricle swabs can be collected for microbiology testing.

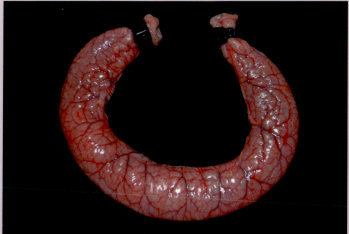

Figure 8. Unopened segments of the intestine with the ends tied off should be submitted for microbiological analysis in case of diarrhoea or presence of enteric lesions.

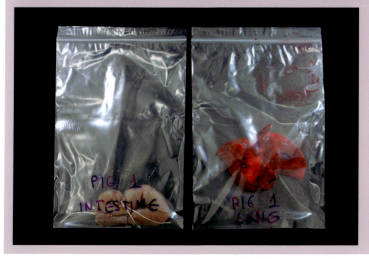

Figure 9. Samples for microbiological studies should be individually packed and identified.

It should be remembered that there is no single toxicology screening that can detect all the known toxic agents. Thus, the choice of toxic substances to be tested in a chemical analysis is based on the clinical, historical, and environmental findings in each case, which will hopefully provide the clinician with a list of potential rule-outs to consider.

Parasitology

Faeces can be submitted for faecal flotation in case of suspicion of intestinal parasites (fig. 10). Fresh or formalin-fixed muscle portions of the tongue, diaphragm, intercostal and masseter muscles should be collected in case of suspicion of muscular parasitosis (trichinosis or cysticercosis). Ear/skin scrapings may be employed to confirm mange (fig. 11).

In some cases, molecular and/or serological techniques have been developed for specific parasitic diseases.

Genetic profiles

Several molecular nucleic acid tests have been developed for genetic testing of different pig diseases (e. g. porcine stress syndrome). In general, blood is the specimen of choice, but the clinician should contact the laboratory for specific genetic tests.

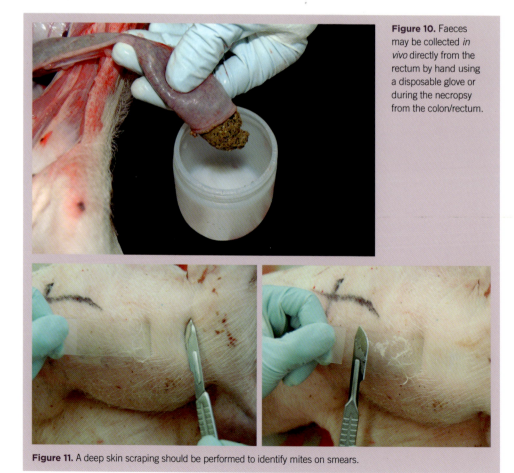

Figure 10. Faeces may be collected *in vivo* directly from the rectum by hand using a disposable glove or during the necropsy from the colon/rectum.

Figure 11. A deep skin scraping should be performed to identify mites on smears.

TABLE 1. Types of samples recommended to be collected at necropsy. These recommendations can be extended for a particular tissue or system depending on the lesions found.

System	Histopathology	Microbiology/virology/PCR	Toxicology	Other
Respiratory	Lung (x2, apical and middle lobes), nasal turbinates	Tissue, swab		
Digestive	Liver, stomach, small intestine (x3, duodenum, jejunum and ileum), large intestine (x2, caecum and colon)	Tissue, swab, saliva	Liver, stomach content, faeces	Faeces (parasitology)
Lympho-hematopoietic	Lymph nodes (x3, i. e., inguinal, mesenteric and mediastinal), tonsil, spleen, bone marrow	Tissue, tonsilar swab		Blood/serum (haematology, biochemistry, genetic profiles)
Urinary	Kidney, urinary bladder	Tissue, swab	Urine	
Cardiovascular	Heart			
Nervous	Brain, spinal cord, trigeminal ganglion	Tissue, swab (meningeal or third ventricle), cerebrospinal fluid	Tissue	
Musculoskeletal	Skeletal muscle (psoas, diaphragm, shoulder, thighs), bone, joint	Swab, tissue		
Integument	Skin (x2)	Tissue, swab	Hair	Scraping (parasitology)
Reproductive	Ovaries, uterus, testicle, mammary gland	Tissue, swab, milk	Milk	
Foetus	Parenchymal organs Placenta	Tissue, swab (stomach content)		

SAMPLING OF AN ANIMAL POPULATION

Often, veterinary surgeons want to know data regarding some specific diseases that can affect pigs on a farm or in a certain region or country. Two main questions can be considered:

1. Is the disease present in the population?
2. What is the proportion (prevalence) of infected animals?

Data collection can be based on the census of the animals (total population) but the selection of an appropriate subsample of animals is simpler and allows time and money saving.

When the objective is to know whether an infection is present or not, data can be collected from animals of the group with more chances of being infected. This is a purposive or convenience sampling method with which the animals are easier to select but may not be representative of the whole population.

To answer the second question, as concerns the prevalence of the infection, the samples have to be representative of the population and must be selected randomly.

FIGURE 12. Flow chart of the sampling process in a population of animals.

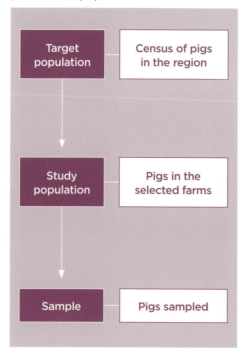

The sampling process entails defining the target (population at risk), the study population (pig farms where the data of the animals will be obtained) and the sample (pigs that will actually be studied) (fig. 12).

The objective of this process is to select a sample of animals whose data can represent the population with an acceptable accuracy, and for this reason two more questions have to be considered:

1. Which individuals have to be included in the sample?
2. How many pigs have to be sampled?

Sampling methods

Probability sampling can be applied to an individual (pig) or to a group (farm) as the sampling units. The most commonly used methods (table 2) in swine epidemiology are the following:

- **Simple random sampling:** every individual from the study population has the same chance of being selected. It can be difficult to apply in practice and is not very efficient.
- **Systematic random sampling:** involves selecting the first pig randomly and the rest of the animals are sampled at regular intervals. This is a very practical method to obtain representative samples from a population.
- **Stratified random sampling:** the population is classified in groups according to a specific factor, for example the age or breed. This is an effective method to reduce variance when a group of animals may be less represented than others in the same population.
- **Cluster sampling:** in this case, the sampling unit is a group of animals that includes individuals that are heterogeneous, while each cluster is similar to the others. Sampling is often clustered by geographical areas, or by time periods.

TABLE 2. Appropriate sampling methods for each type and characteristics of a pig population.

Characteristics of population	Type of population	Appropriate sampling method
Homogeneous	Fattening pigs/slaughterhouse	Simple random/systematic random
Different strata (age, breed, number of animals) but homogeneous within strata	Farrow-to-finish farms, stratified by age Farms stratified by number of sows	Stratified sampling
Similar regions (country), with heterogeneous farms within them	Group of farms in selected regions	Cluster sampling

Sample size

The number of pigs to be sampled depends on the objective of the sampling.

A. Sampling to **determine the prevalence** of an infection or disease in the population. The factors to take into consideration are:

- The expected frequency of the infection (p); i.e. a hypothesis on the proportion of infected animals (example: $p = 20\%$).
- The accuracy or level of precision required (B); it means the distance of the sample estimate that is acceptable (example: $B = \pm 5\%$).
- The desired confidence level; usually 90-95-99%, for a distribution of the population to be normal. The corresponding standard errors (z) are 1.65-1.96-2.58 (example: 95% and $z = 1.96$).
- Number of animals in the population (N).

Then, the formula to calculate sample size (n) to determine prevalence is:

$$n = \frac{z^2 p (1 - p)}{B^2} \blacktriangleright n = \frac{1.96 * 0.20 (0.80)}{0.05^2} = 246$$

For small populations, the calculated sample size (n) may be too high, and the total

number of animals (N) has to be considered to estimate an adjusted sample size (n'):

$$\frac{1}{n'} = \frac{1}{n} + \frac{1}{N} \overset{N = 500 \text{ pigs}}{\blacktriangleright} \frac{1}{n'} = \frac{1}{246} + \frac{1}{500} \blacktriangleright n' = 165$$

These calculations can easily be made by means of epidemiology computer programmes such as Winepi (http://www.winepi.net) or FreeCalc (http://www.ausvet.com.au/content.php?page=software#freecalc), or by using tables. An example of sample size calculation for a 95% confidence level and different values of accuracy and expected prevalence can be found in table 3.

B. Sampling to **detect the presence of a disease**, regardless of the proportion of infected animals. This calculation is useful in outbreak investigations, disease control or eradication programmes. The aim is to calculate the sample size needed to know whether the disease is present or not in the population (N), considering a desired confidence level (a, in percentage) and the number of infected animals in case the disease is present (D).

$$n = [1 - (1 - a)^{1/D}] * [N - ((D - 1)/2)]$$

The use of tables or computer programmes can simplify this calculation (table 4). For example, if the expected disease prevalence is 10% and the population size is 500 animals, a sample of 28 pigs is required to be 95% certain of detecting at least one diseased pig. If among all the selected animals, none is sick, the interpretation is that the disease is not present at that expected prevalence or that if it exists, the prevalence is lower than 10%.

TABLE 3. Sample size to determine prevalence with 95% confidence level.

Prevalence	Desired precision (accuracy)						
	25%	20%	10%	5%	3%	1%	0.5%
5%	3	5	19	73	292	1,825	7,300
10%	6	9	35	139	554	3,458	13,830
15%	8	13	49	196	784	4,899	19,593
20%	10	16	62	246	984	6,147	24,857
25%	12	19	73	289	1,153	7,203	28,812
30%	13	21	81	323	1,291	8,068	32,270
35%	14	22	88	350	1,399	8,740	34,959
40%	15	24	93	369	1,476	9,220	36,880
45%	16	24	96	381	1,522	9,508	38,032
50%	16	25	97	385	1,537	9,604	38,416

TABLE 4. Sample size to detect presence of disease with a 95% confidence level.

Number of animals	Expected prevalence if the disease is present								
	90%	80%	70%	60%	50%	40%	30%	20%	10%
5	2	2	3	3	3	3	5	5	5
10	2	2	3	3	4	4	6	8	10
12	2	2	3	4	4	5	7	9	11
15	2	2	3	4	5	5	7	9	13
20	2	2	3	4	5	6	7	10	19
30	2	2	3	4	5	6	8	11	19
50	2	2	3	4	5	6	8	12	22
80	2	2	3	4	5	6	9	13	24
100	2	2	3	4	5	6	9	13	25
200	2	2	3	4	5	6	9	14	27
500	2	2	3	4	5	6	9	14	28
1,000	2	2	3	4	5	6	9	14	29

3

Submission of samples for laboratory diagnosis

The quality and value of laboratory results directly depend on the proper collection, submission and processing of samples. Consequently, taking the right precautions at the time of collecting and transporting the sample is critical for a reliable diagnosis (figs. 1-5).

Based on the clinical suspicion and the type of analytical test, the samples can be collected for different diagnostic purposes (table 1).

The submission of a sample has to be accompanied by a submission form. This information is crucial in those cases in which the laboratory personnel are expected to give an interpretation of the results. The minimum information the report should include is the following:

- Date of sampling.
- Sample reference (identification number).
- Identification of the owner/company (contact details).
- Origin of the sample (animal species, physiological characteristics).
- Type of sample.
- Clinical background of the animal/farm: farm population, type of management

(farrowing, growing, finishing, etc.), past or current diseases.
- Description of the current problem: affected ages, symptoms, duration, morbidity and mortality rates.
- Treatments (historical and current): vaccination, antibiotics.
- Clinical suspicion.
- Analytical request.

An example of an application form is shown in figure 6.

Depending on the nature of the clinical signs and origin of the sample, the procedure of collection and submission for laboratory diagnosis may not always be the same (table 2).

For pathologic studies, a similar clinical history is required. If field necropsy is performed, a report of gross findings is recommended. Describe any organic abnormality: colour, consistency, size and shape. Macroscopic diagnoses are also useful (e. g. fibrinous pleuritis, ulcerative enteritis) but it is important to describe the distribution (focal, focally extensive, multifocal, diffuse) and severity (mild, moderate, severe) of the lesions.

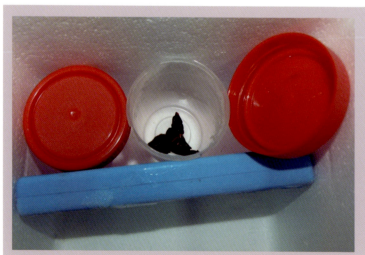

Figure 1. For microbiological analyses, the samples must be sent individually (not mixed with others), in a sterile, airtight container or bag and kept refrigerated.

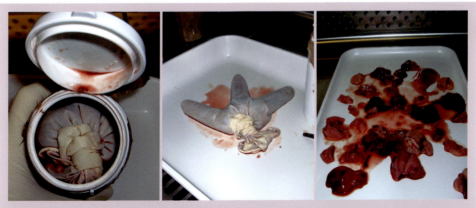

Figure 2. Examples of incorrect sample submission for microbiological (bacteriological/mycological) diagnosis. On the left, a container with a glove full of samples appears dirty and externally contaminated with exudates from the samples. In the middle, a more detailed picture of the glove containing the samples. On the right, the samples from different organs that were found in the glove.

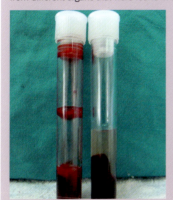

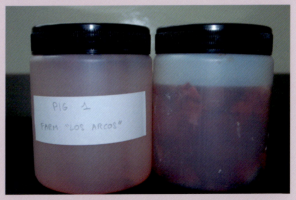

Figure 3. For serological analyses, the serum has to be separated from the whole blood. The collection tubes must not contain any anticoagulants to allow clot formation. The serum should be transparent (right) and with no signs of haemolysis or putrefaction (left).

Figure 4. For histopathological examination, the left plastic jar is an example of correct sample submission: the jar is correctly identified and contains a large proportion of formalin. However, the right jar is an example of incorrect submission: the jar is not labelled, has a small quantity of formalin in relation to the amount of tissue and the samples are too large (difficult/delayed formalin fixation).

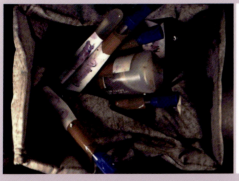

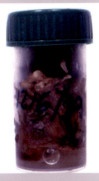

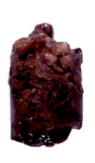

Figure 5. Two examples of incorrect sample submission for histopathological examination. On the left, a glass jar was broken during its shipment causing formalin leakage and the ink of the labels to run. On the right, a small jar with an insufficient proportion of formalin and a portion of tissue that is too large caused incorrect fixation and autolysis of the samples.

TABLE 1. Characteristics and key points of sample submission for the different laboratory diagnoses.

Diagnosis	Basis	Critical points
Bacteriology/ Mycology	Isolation and identification of bacteria or fungal pathogens.	■ Asepsis (sterile containers and instruments for taking the sample). ■ Cooling at 4 °C (no freezing or fixing with formalin). ■ Sterile handling and submission of all the viscera (figs. 1 and 2). ■ Fresh samples (< 12-24 h). ■ No antimicrobial (parenteral) treatment of the animal at least 2 days before sampling.
Virology	Isolation of virus and detection of virus or viral antigens (IF, IPMA).	■ Asepsis (sterile containers and instruments for taking the sample). ■ Cooling at 4 °C or freezing (no fixing with formalin). ■ Fresh samples (< 24 h).
Serology	Detection of antibodies (indirect, direct or competitive ELISA) or antigens (capture or sandwich ELISA) in serum.	■ Aseptic bleeding preferred. ■ Sterile and airtight syringes or tubes. ■ No anticoagulants. ■ Separation of the serum from the coagulum is preferred. ■ Cooling (4 °C) or at room temperature (can be frozen if serum). ■ Remove needles. ■ Submission in appropriate containers to avoid tube ruptures (fig. 3).
Histopathology	Identification and description of lesions. Identification of pathogens (IHC, ISH).	■ Fixed samples in containers with 10% buffered formalin (figs. 4 and 5). ■ Use small sections of organs to ensure complete fixation. ■ Submission at room temperature. ■ Minimum fixation time of 24 h. ■ Airtight containers.
Molecular Biology	Detection of genetic components (PCR).	■ Fresh or frozen samples to avoid degradation (mainly for RNA). ■ Submission of the entire organ is preferred. ■ Selection of the target organs (to ensure presence of pathogens).
Parasitology	Detection and identification of parasites.	■ Cooling 4 °C (no freezing or fixing with formalin). ■ Fresh samples (< 12-24 h). ■ Submission of viscera with parasitic lesions.
Toxicology	Detection of toxics.	■ Having a suspicious diagnosis of a toxic substance or poison.

TABLE 2. Types of samples, sample-taking procedure and shipment timing for laboratory submission, according to clinical symptoms.

Clinical problem	Sample	Sample taking procedure	Time between sample taking and reception at the laboratory
Respiratory symptoms	a) Lungs, nasal turbinates b) Tracheo-bronchial lavage c) Nasal swabs*	a) At necropsy. b and c) Living animals. This requires restraining the animal. Maximise asepsis as the sample can easily be contaminated (b). c) Not recommended for microbiological isolation (highly contaminated).	12 h/24 h**
Digestive/enteric symptoms	a) Intestine b) Faeces	a) At necropsy. Submission of the small and large intestines with the faeces and both ends tied off. b) Living animals. Collection of clean faeces from the rectum (avoid faeces from the soil).	a) 12 h/24 h b) 24 h/48 h
Nervous symptoms	a) Brain, meningeal swabs* b) Cerebrospinal fluid	At necropsy.	12 h
Systemic symptoms	Viscera	At necropsy. Liver and spleen. Other organs with gross lesions.	12 h/24 h
Otitis, conjunctivitis	Inner ear and ocular swabs*	Clean the anatomical region before collecting the sample.	12 h/24 h
Cystitis	Urine	a) Cystocentesis. This is the most aseptic method. b) Catheterisation. Previously clean the penile/vulvar region. c) Spontaneous urination. Discard the first streams of urine.	6 h
Mastitis	Milk from all mammary glands	Udder wash and disinfection. Discard the first streams of milk. Collect samples from all glands.	12 h
Abortions/reproductive symptoms	a) Foetuses b) Vaginal secretion	a) Protection with mask and gloves and avoid excessive manipulation (zoonotic risk). Send foetus together with placenta if possible. b) Use swabs and clean the genital region before collecting the sample.	12 h/24 h
Skin problems (pyodermas)	a) Epidermal/dermal scraping b) Hair	a) Scrape deeply around the skin lesions with sterile scalpel blades. b) Remove the skin, mainly for mycotic isolation.	24 h/48 h

*Sterile cotton swabs with transport medium are preferred in all cases.
**12 h during hot seasons and 24 h during cold periods.

FIGURE 6. Example of a request form for different laboratory diagnostic tests.

Submission Form
for laboratory diagnosis

Case N°
(laboratory number)

Company:
Veterinary surgeon:
Farm/Reference:
Region:
Contact telephone number:
Fax/e-mail:
Date of sample collection:
Date of sample remittance:

(to be completed by the lab)

Arrival date:
Supervisor:

Sample data

Species:
Age:

Submitted sample (type and number)

Received samples (to be completed by the lab)

Background and current clinical signs/recent relevant treatments

Analyses required

IMMUNOLOGICAL DIAGN.
- [ ] PRRSV
- [ ] ADV gE
- [ ] ADV total Abs
- [ ] Porcine parvovirus
- [ ] *E. rhusiopathiae*
- [ ] Swine influenza virus
- [ ] *M. hyopneumoniae*
- [ ] Toxigenic *Pasteurella* spp.
- [ ] *A. pleuropneumoniae*
- [ ] *Salmonella* spp.
- [ ] Immunoglobulin quantification
- [ ] Others (please specify)

MOLECULAR DIAGN.
- [ ] PCR PRRS (European strains)
- [ ] PCR PRRS (American strains)
- [ ] PCR *P. multocida* (toxigenic strains)
- [ ] PCR Swine influenza
- [ ] PCR *M. hyopneumoniae*
- [ ] PCR *B. hyodysenteriae*
- [ ] PCR *B. pilosicoli*
- [ ] PCR *L. intracellularis*
- [ ] PCR PCV1
- [ ] PCR PCV2

MICROBIOLOGICAL DIAGN.
- [ ] General isolation and identification
- [ ] Isolation and identification of respiratory pathogens
- [ ] Isolation and identification of enteric pathogens
- [ ] Specific isolation of:
  - [ ] Antibiogram
  - [ ] Minimum inhibitory concentration
  - [ ] *E. coli* quantification
  - [ ] Others (please specify)

OTHERS
- [ ] Vaccine titration
- [ ] Seroneutralisation test

Observations

Note: reverse side can be used for additional information.

4

Diagnostic methods

HISTOPATHOLOGICAL TECHNIQUES

Pathological analysis is a very commonly used tool for the laboratory diagnosis of swine diseases. In some cases, several pigs are submitted to the laboratory for their necropsy and subsequent histopathological analysis. However, in other cases, the veterinary surgeon performs an on-farm necropsy and submits formalin-fixed tissues or other fresh samples to the laboratory (see chapters 2 and 3).

Pathological analyses consist of the identification and description of the lesions present in the animals (figs. 1, 2 and 3). In many cases, the morphological changes observed in the animal tissues, together with the results of the microbiological, molecular, parasitological or serological analyses are rather indicative of the aetiology of the disorder. On some occasions, the pathologist needs to use other histological techniques to identify the causative agent.

Special stains such as the Ziehl-Neelsen stain for mycobacteria, periodic acid-Schiff (PAS) and Grocott's methenamine silver stains (fig. 4) for fungi or yeast, or the Warthin-Starry silver stain (fig. 5) for spirochetes are, for example, used to detect certain specific infectious agents in tissues. Nevertheless, most of the infectious agents involved in the appearance of lesions are not identified with special stains and it is necessary to use other techniques.

Immunohistochemistry (IHC) is a useful technique to detect antigens or proteins in tissue sections by means of specific antibodies (figs. 6 and 7). The range of proteins that are possible to detect is very broad and includes infectious agents (viruses, bacteria, parasites, fungi, protozoa, yeast and prions), tumoral markers, specific proteins (amyloid) and cell receptors. Specific cell events such as proliferation or cell death (apoptosis) can also be detected. The advantage of IHC is that it has a high specificity and moderate sensitivity, but it is more time-consuming and expensive than special stains. Once the antigen-antibody binding occurs, the positive result is demonstrated with a coloured histochemical reaction visible by light microscopy or fluorochromes with ultraviolet light. Although it can be performed on frozen tissue, formalin-fixed tissues are most commonly used for this technique in routine laboratory diagnosis.

In situ hybridisation is another specific technique used to detect DNA or RNA of specific infectious agents in tissue sections. It is described in the section about molecular biology techniques later in this chapter.

BACTERIOLOGICAL TECHNIQUES

The main objective of bacteriological diagnosis is the isolation and identification of bacteria involved in pathological processes, according to their ability to grow on various selective media, the characteristic appearance of their colonies and their ability to react when biochemical tests are used. The efficient use and correct interpretation of clinical bacteriology analyses can be a helpful tool in the diagnosis of some infectious diseases.

Basic techniques in bacteriological diagnosis

The first step in a bacteriological analysis is to make a smear of fresh samples or swabs on a clean slide and stain it to observe under a microscope for bacteria. The potential type of organism should be identified and its relative amount estimated. This is useful to decide which culture media and conditions have to be used for a tentative isolation.

The Gram stain (Box 1) remains the most frequently used rapid diagnostic test and is one of the bases of clinical laboratory practice together with biochemical tests.

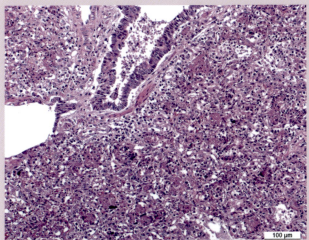

Figure 1. Lung, haematoxylin-eosin stain. Marked presence of necrotic cell clusters in the alveoli in a case of proliferative and neocrotising pneumonia. This pathological condition has been related with PRRSV and PCV2, although its pathogenesis is unknown.

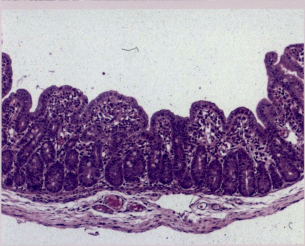

Figure 2. Small intestine, haematoxylin-eosin stain. Severe atrophy and fusion of the intestinal villi in the jejunum. This lesion can be caused by a number of organisms such as coccidian protozoa, viruses (coronavirus and rotavirus) and bacteria (*Escherichia coli*). This particular case was caused by the virus of transmissible gastroenteritis (TGEV).

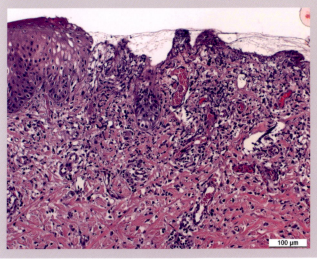

Figure 3. Skin, haematoxylin-eosin stain. Cutaneous ulceration with superficial dermis inflammation and necrosis; the epidermal margin show keratinocytes with ballooning degeneration typical of swine poxvirus infection.

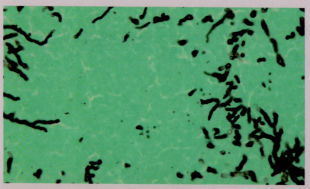

Figure 4. Lung, Grocott staining. Presence of *Aspergillus* spp. Hyphae (black staining) showing uniformity in width, septation and acutely angled, dichotomous branching in the lumen of a bronchus filled with necrotic inflammatory cells. This animal was concomitantly suffering from porcine circovirus type 2-systemic disease.

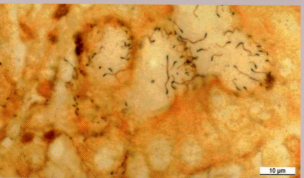

Figure 5. Colon, Warthin-Starry silver stain. Presence of spirochete bacteria (black spiral-shaped filaments) in the colon mucosa of a pig with bloody-mucous diarrhoea. Although the technique cannot establish the precise aetiology of the disease, these microorganisms are highly suggestive of *Brachyspira hyodysenteriae*.

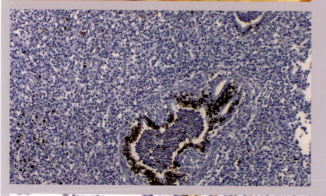

Figure 6.
Lung, immunohistochemistry to detect the swine influenza virus. High amount of SIV antigen (brown staining) in the epithelial cells of a bronchus, as well as sporadic presence of the antigen in some alveolar macrophages in the inflammatory infiltrates of the lung parenchyma.

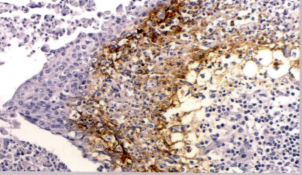

Figure 7.
Tonsil, immunohistochemistry to detect the Aujeszky's disease virus (ADV) or pseudorabies virus (PRV). Presence of ADV antigen (brown staining) located in the necrotic focus of the tonsil.

BOX 1. Brief summary of the steps to perform a Gram stain technique on a smear.

Gram stain technique
1. Air dry specimen and fix with methanol or heat.
2. Add crystal violet stain (30–60 sec.)
3. Rinse with water to wash unbound dye, add mordant (30–60 sec.) (for example, iodine: potassium iodide).
4. Add decolouriser (ethanol or acetone) to remove unbound dye.
5. Counterstain with safranin or fucsine (60 sec.).
6. Rinse with water.
Gram-positive bacteria stain blue (retained crystal violet). Gram-negative bacteria stain red (decolourised and then counterstained).

In some cases, it may be interesting to observe fresh samples using a phase contrast microscope, for example when the presence of *Brachyspira* spp. or *Leptospira* spp. is suspected, because in these cases, specific media and incubation conditions are needed to obtain successful results.

One of the primary diagnostic methods is bacteriological culture. Different agar media are used to grow and identify the type of organism responsible for -or that is a component of- a given infectious disease. Depending on the clinical suspicion, the samples are inoculated in a Petri dish with an enriched medium (blood agar, chocolate agar), a differential medium (McConkey agar) or both. Selective media are also used for the isolation of specific microorganisms (XLT4 agar to grow *Salmonella* spp. from faeces, for example).

Moreover, enriched broth cultures are used when the animals have been treated with antibiotics before sampling and only a small amount of the organism may be available in the sample.

For routine purposes, the inoculated plates and culture broth are incubated at 37 °C aerobically for 24 hours, but longer periods of time and lower or higher temperatures of incubation may be needed. In addition, anaerobic (e. g. *Clostridium* spp.) or microaerophilic (e. g *Haemophilus* spp.) cultures are used for the growth of selected organisms; these special conditions may be used on demand, when there is a suspicion of a causative agent, and some laboratories use them on a routine basis.

Bacterial identification

A standardised protocol of identification includes the following steps:

1. **Morphological and Gram identification**: type, colour and morphology of the colonies grown on the agar medium, e. g. grey mucoid colonies of *Pasteurella multocida*, small white colonies of *Streptococcus suis* and swarming growth of *Proteus* spp. on blood agar. Moreover, the Gram stain of the selected colonies allows the classification of the bacteria as cocci/bacilli, positive/negative.

Other features to consider:
- **Capacity to lyse erythrocytes**: haemolysis in blood agar is usually considered to determine the virulence of certain strains, such as *Escherichia coli*, or to identify certain *Streptococcus* spp. However, it

is important to note that although the presence of haemolysins synthesised by a certain strain is indicative of virulence, there are many other factors that can indicate virulence. Thus, if an abundant pure culture of non-haemolytic *E. coli* is isolated from the faeces of a pig suffering from a diarrheal process, *E. coli* can be considered the aetiological agent despite the lack of haemolysis. Different degrees of haemolysis can be found in blood agar: no haemolysis (γ-haemolysis), incomplete haemolysis (α-haemolysis) associated with a reduction of red cell haemoglobin, and complete haemolysis (β-haemolysis) (fig. 8).

- **Colony recounts:** the number of colony-forming units, usually abbreviated as CFU, refers to individual colonies of bacteria, yeast or mould. The quantification of the number of colonies that grow in a culture can be used to determine the actual involvement in a pathological process of bacteria that are common in the

saprophytic flora (e. g. enteritis caused by non-haemolytic *E. coli* strains).
2. **Biochemical characterisation** (in-house test or commercial API tests).
3. **Immunological characterisation** by means of the use of specific antisera for serotyping *Salmonella* spp. or *E. coli*.
4. **Molecular characterisation** (PCR, hybridisation methods); see the specific part on molecular biology diagnostic methods in this chapter.

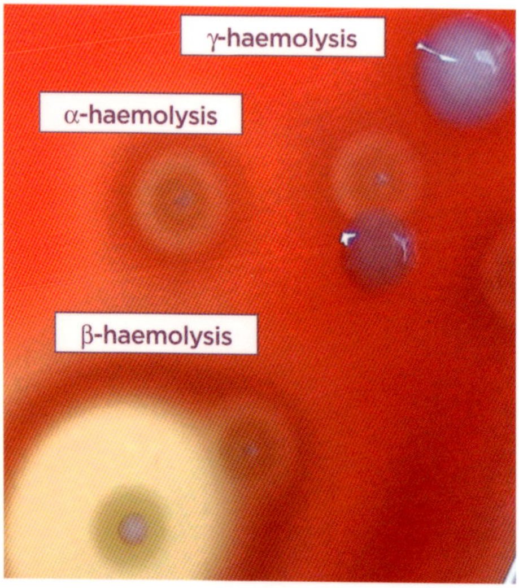

A flow chart to identify bacterial pathogens by means of Gram stain and biochemical profiles is shown in figures 9a and 9b.

Methods to determine antimicrobial activity

One of the most practical pieces of information provided by the clinical bacteriology laboratory to veterinary practitioners is the antimicrobial activity of bacterial isolates, which allows the selection of an appropriate treatment. Moreover, the clinical bacteriology laboratory can offer methods that allow greater precision in the diagnosis and, as a result, a reduction of the use of inappropriate antibiotics and of the selection of antimicrobial resistant strains.

One of the main applications of clinical bacteriology is the antibiogram. This technique is defined as a laboratory method in which a pure isolate of bacteria is treated with a variety of antibiotics in order to determine its antimicrobial susceptibility or resistance *in vitro*. There are two different procedures to assess antimicrobial resistance:

A. **Kirby-Bauer method** (or disc diffusion antibiotic sensitivity testing): it is a qualitative method that involves using small discs containing different antibiotics in known concentrations in a bacterial culture on a nutrient-rich agar medium (fig. 10). The antibiotic will diffuse around each tablet

γ-haemolysis

α-haemolysis

β-haemolysis

Figure 8. Bacterial colonies with different degrees of haemolysis in a blood agar medium.

FIGURE 9a. Flow chart to identify bacterial pathogens with a Gram stain and biochemical profiles. Gram-negative bacteria.

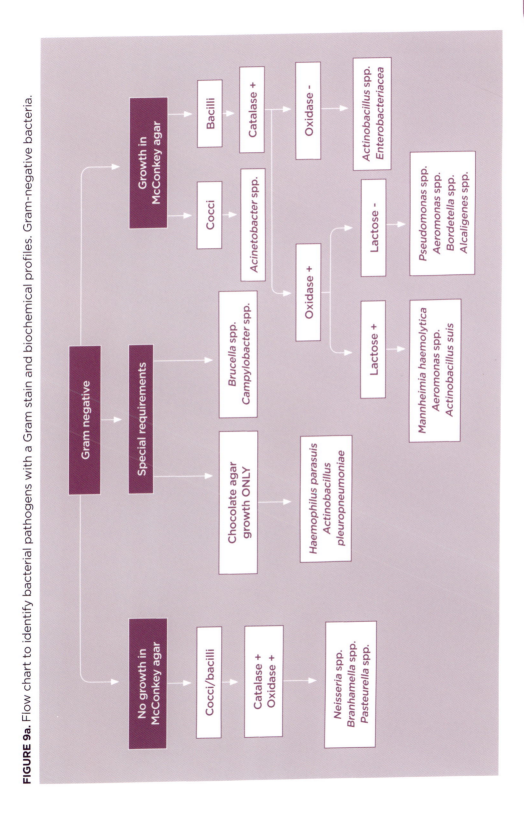

FIGURE 9b. Flow chart to identify bacterial pathogens with a Gram stain and biochemical profiles. Gram-positive bacteria.

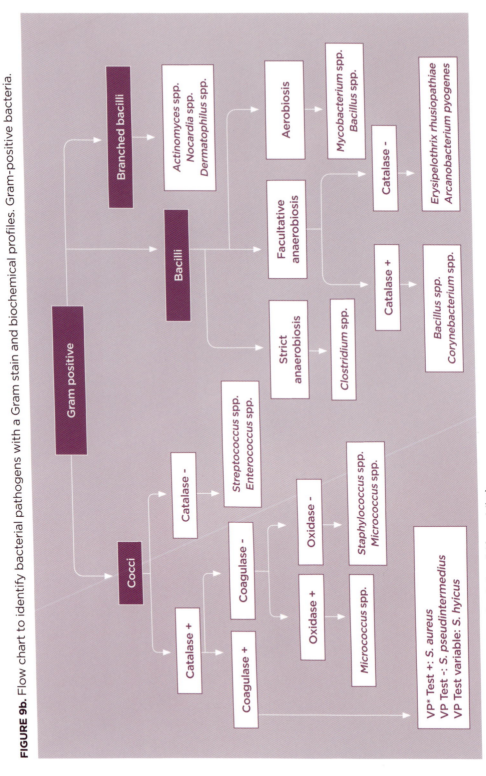

*VP Test: Voges-Proskauer (determines butanediol fermentation).

and an area of bacterial growth inhibition will appear. Thus, the diameter is suggestive of the antimicrobial susceptibility of the bacteria and the interpretation is made based on international standards. A bacterial strain can be reported as susceptible, intermediate or resistant to a certain antibiotic. This method is one of the most routinely used in laboratory practice due to its fast and simple application.

B. **Minimal Inhibitory Concentration (MIC)**: it is a quantitative method reported as micrograms per millilitre (µg/ml), which represents the lowest drug concentration that prevents visible microorganism growth after overnight incubation with the corresponding media. The microbroth dilution method, one of the most commonly used ones, involves introducing the same amount of bacteria into different wells containing a liquid medium with progressively lower concentrations of the tested drug. This procedure is more precise than the Kirby-Bauer method but it is more time-consuming and laborious.

The use of the MIC may be interesting for veterinary surgeons, to treat animals with specific infections, as it can help in the selection of the most appropriate antibiotic and at an effective dose. This latter aspect is crucial because the populations of bacteria exposed to an insufficient concentration of a determined drug or to a broad-spectrum antibiotic can become resistant to these drugs. In general, in cases where the efficacy of the antimicrobial treatment has to be enhanced or the selection of antimicrobial-resistant strains minimised, the use of the MIC is recommended.

Interpretation of results

For a correct interpretation of bacteriological results, it is crucial to identify the following elements:

- The normal saprophytic flora existing in the sample.
- Contaminating bacteria (species of the Enterobacteriaceae family, *Pseudomonas* spp., *Staphylococcus* spp.) originated from incorrect manipulation of the sample or environmental contamination.
- Significance of the obtained isolate regarding the suspected aetiology and its role as a primary or secondary agent; this significance must be established by the submitting veterinary surgeon and, in case of doubts, it is recommended to contact the diagnostic laboratory.

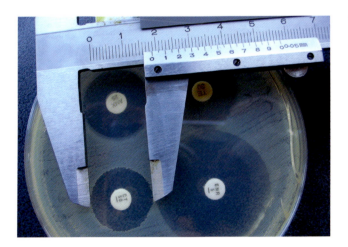

Figure 10. Antibiogram showing different areas of susceptibility and resistance for a particular *E. coli* isolate, using the Kirby–Bauer method.

VIROLOGICAL TECHNIQUES

The main objective of virological diagnosis is the identification of a viral aetiology potentially involved in a pathological process. The methodology followed in the laboratory is based on one of the following principles:

- Identification of viral particles by electron microscopy (EM). The distinct morphology and size of the particles allows their classification into a family of viruses, e. g. herpesvirus, coronavirus, influenza, circovirus, rotavirus, etc. However, EM is relatively insensitive and requires specific equipment. This is why EM is not included in routine procedures.
- Detection of viral antigens in infected tissues or secretions. Their detection is based on specific antigen-antibody reactions and is done using mainly capture-ELISA, immunofluorescence and/or immunoperoxidase tests.
- Isolation of a virus in a cell culture or another living host (tissues, organ cultures or experimental animals). This is the most specific and sensitive procedure, but several days or weeks are necessary to confirm or rule out a viral infection.
- Detection of viral nucleic acids by PCR or DNA hybridisation (see molecular biology section).
- Demonstration of specific antibody titres (see serology section).

Basic techniques in virological diagnosis

Virus isolation consists of two steps: the recovery of the virus and identification of the isolate. Isolation is usually attempted by means of *in vitro* cell cultures. The identification of the isolate is done using immunofluorescence, electron microscopy or molecular techniques.

- **Virus isolation**: Viruses are obligate intracellular parasites that require living cells in order to replicate. There are many biological media that can be used to isolate viruses (table 1).
- **Viral identification**: Several laboratory tests are used to detect the presence of a viral agent. One of the most common methods is the assessment of cellular alterations caused by viral replication in the cellular medium, known as cytopathogenic effect (CPE). As only some virus can induce visible CPE, there are other methods that help to identify the viral agent by detecting specific proteins or genomic compounds of the virus (fig. 11).

The isolation and identification of a specific virus in sick animals is considered to be a definitive diagnosis. However, these procedures are frequently laborious (qualified staff is required), expensive (sterile material and special facilities), and time consuming (results available after 1-2 weeks of sample processing). Therefore, viral isolation should mainly be considered when the isolate is required for antigenic or genetic characterisation, and other virological approaches or applications.

Virological identification includes the following steps:

1. **Presumptive identification:**
   - Susceptibility of culture cells to viruses.
   - CPE observed (fig. 12).
   - Haemadsorption: viruses with haemagglutinins in their envelope such as influenza viruses, paramyxoviruses or asfiviruses.
2. **Definitive identification:** using specific assays to detect viral proteins or nucleic acid:
   - **Immunofluorescence (IF)**: this assay is based on the fluorescence emitted by virus-specific antibodies labelled

TABLE 1. Description of the different biological media for virus isolation.

Biological medium		Use	Limitations
Cell cultures	Primary cell cultures	▪ Isolation of virus not adapted to immortalised cell lines.	▪ Limited cell life (5-10 cell division cycles). ▪ Requires continuous collection from donors.
	Semi-continuous cells: foetal origin	▪ Isolation of some viruses that do not grow in continuous cell lines.	▪ Limited cell life (up to 50-100 cellular divisions).
	Continuous cell lines: tumour cells	▪ Common viral isolation diagnosis and research. ▪ Cheap and fast method. ▪ Large production of cells (unlimited cell division).	▪ Some viruses cannot replicate and thus cannot be isolated because a previous viral adaptation in cell lines is needed.
Chicken embryo eggs		▪ For primary isolation of influenza virus and others. ▪ Epidemiological studies and vaccine production.	▪ Time consuming. ▪ Laborious. ▪ Expensive. ▪ High quality eggs (high health status).
Laboratory animals		▪ When none of the other options is available. ▪ For research purposes.	▪ Working with live animals (expensive, time-consuming, trained staff, animal welfare guidelines).

with a fluorochrome, usually fluorescein. The specific complexes of a viral antigen and a labelled antibody appear as fluorescent green spots under ultraviolet radiation. It can be performed on frozen tissue sections or cell cultures but, for better results, frozen tissue sections require fresh clinical specimens (fig. 13).

- **Immunohistochemistry (IHC)**: antigen detection method used on formalin-fixed tissues. This assay utilises virus-specific antibodies labelled with an enzyme, mainly peroxidase (see histopathology section).

- **Virus neutralisation:** this neutralisation test is based on the principle that a live virus will be neutralised by its specific antibody and will thus be unable to infect susceptible cells.

- **Haemadsorption, haemagglutination and haemagglutination inhibition**: the haemadsorption test is based on the fact that pig erythrocytes will adhere to the surface of cells infected with certain viruses, such as asfivirus (ASFV). On the other hand, the haemagglutinating capacity of some viruses such as the influenza viruses can be blocked by a specific antibody, thus inhibiting the agglutination of erythrocytes (fig. 14).

- **Electron microscopy**: mostly for research purposes.

- **Antigen-capture ELISA**: this assay allows the detection of viruses or viral antigens in clinical samples using two

FIGURE 11. Steps of the general procedure for virus isolation.

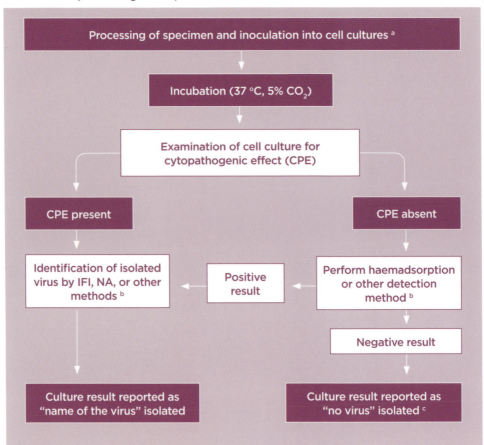

[a] Cell lines such as PK-15 (PCV2), MARC-145 (PRRSV), MDCK and Vero cells
    (porcine rubulavirus, swine influenza virus).
[b] Indirect immunofluorescence (IFI), neutralisation assays (NA), enzyme immunoassay (IPMA),
    nucleic acid probe, complement fixation and haemaglutination inhibition assays.
[c] If viruses do not proliferate in conventional cell lines, other methods such as alternative culture systems
    (primary cells tissues, eggs, experimental animals) can be applied.

different specific antibodies to capture the virus present in the sample. The antigen-capture ELISA is a variant of the indirect ELISA test to detect antibodies (see serological techniques, fig. 22a), but in this case a variety of clinical samples, such as fluid, saliva, excretions, plasma, tissue or faecal suspension, can be used for diagnosis. This technique is faster and cheaper and its sensitivity is sufficient compared to other virological techniques. It is used as a routine diagnostic method in many laboratories.

- **Molecular techniques such as PCR or DNA hybridisation** (see molecular biology section).

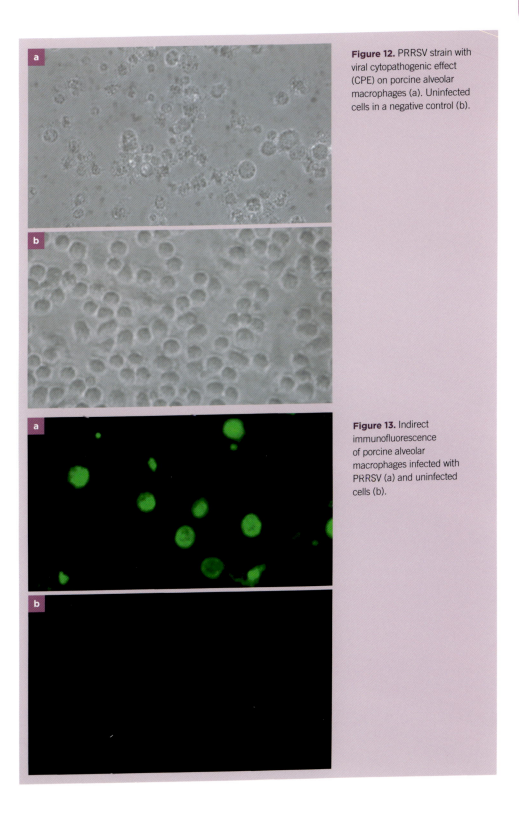

Figure 12. PRRSV strain with viral cytopathogenic effect (CPE) on porcine alveolar macrophages (a). Uninfected cells in a negative control (b).

Figure 13. Indirect immunofluorescence of porcine alveolar macrophages infected with PRRSV (a) and uninfected cells (b).

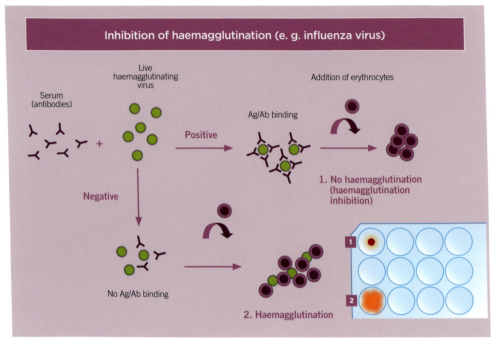

Figure 14. Haemagglutination inhibition testing. In the first stage, the haemagglutinating viruses and the serum with the antibodies are mixed. In a second stage, erythrocytes are added. If the serum contains virus-specific antibodies (positive sample), these bind to the virus and the virus fails to haemagglutinate the erythrocytes. If the sample does not contain any specific antibodies (negative sample), the virus remains active and haemagglutinates the erythrocytes. Haemagglutination appears as a shield of tiny aggregates at the bottom of the well. Non-agglutinated cells settle in the centre of the well. Ag: antigen; Ab: antibody.

MOLECULAR BIOLOGY TECHNIQUES

This section provides the general principles of the molecular techniques commonly used as diagnostic tools in swine diseases, as well as some of their practical applications.

Principles of molecular techniques

Molecular diagnosis assays are based on the detection of a specific nucleic acid segment (DNA or RNA) in a test specimen. In the particular case of swine diseases, those tools are used to detect infectious agents. Test specimens may be swabs, body fluids, blood, serum, stool or tissues.

The main molecular diagnostic techniques to detect or quantify the presence of a pathogen in a given sample are listed below (table 2):

- **Polymerase chain reaction (PCR)**: it is a rapid diagnostic test to detect DNA of a suspected pathogen within a sample. The key component of the PCR is a pair of short specific DNA fragments, called primers, complementary to the target DNA. This laboratory method is based on three steps: DNA extraction, amplification and detection (agarose gel electrophoresis).
- **Nested PCR (nPCR)**: it is a modification of the abovementioned PCR, since it uses a second pair of primers (located within the first pair of primers) and a second round of amplification. This modification

TABLE 2. Characteristics of the main molecular diagnostic techniques to detect or quantify the presence of a pathogen in a given sample.

Technique	Target	Key components	Visualisation of results	Interpretation of results
PCR	DNA	Primers, DNA polymerase	Electrophoresis (agarose gel)	Positive or negative
nPCR	DNA	Outer and inner primers, DNA polymerase	Electrophoresis (agarose gel)	Positive or negative
RT-PCR	RNA	Reverse-transcriptase, primers, DNA polymerase	Electrophoresis (agarose gel)	Positive or negative
Multiplex PCR	DNA	Different primers pairs, DNA polymerase	Electrophoresis (agarose gel)	Positive or negative
qPCR	DNA	Primers, DNA polymerase and specific or non-specific dye	Fluorescence	Positive or negative Amount of pathogen
RT-qPCR	RNA	Reverse-transcriptase, primers, DNA polymerase and specific or non-specific dye	Fluorescence	Positive or negative Amount of pathogen
ISH	DNA/RNA	Probe	Fluorescence or optical microscopy	Positive or negative (in tissue)

provides a higher sensitivity. Nested PCR is used in those pathologies in which the amount of target DNA in the samples is very limited.

- **Reverse-transcriptase PCR (RT-PCR):** method to detect RNA. It includes the same three basic parts of the PCR, with an additional step using a reverse-transcriptase enzyme to synthesise complementary DNA from the target RNA. The complementary DNA is then amplified with the conventional PCR technique.
- **Multiplex PCR:** it consists in the detection of several DNA/RNA fragments by means

of the use of multiple primer sets in a single PCR reaction.

- **Quantitative, real time PCR (qPCR):** it simultaneously amplifies and quantifies the amount of DNA after each PCR cycle. Its key feature is the presence of a specific dye (probe) located between the pair of primers, or non-specific fluorescent dyes that bind to any double-stranded DNA. It is based on the detection and quantification of the fluorescence emitted by the specific or non-specific dye. The pathogen load is calculated by means of an extrapolation from a standard curve.

- **RT-qPCR**: it is a qPCR test with a previous step including the transcription from RNA to DNA.
- *In situ* **hybridisation (ISH)**: it is based on the detection of specific complementary sequences of nucleic acids present in a tissue using labelled nucleic acid sequences (probes). The hybridisation is revealed by an enzymatic reaction or by the emission of light by a fluorochrome.

There are several molecular techniques to determine the different genotypes of a pathogen present in a diagnostic specimen. Some of the methods used for genotyping are PCR, genome sequencing, restriction fragment length polymorphism identification (RFLPI), random amplification of polymorphic DNA (RAPD), amplified fragment length polymorphism detection (AFLP) and hybridisation to DNA microarrays or beads. These genotyping methods are used to determine the DNA sequence of a given pathogen present in a diagnostic specimen and to compare it with other reference sequences/patrons. This information will be used to identify the epidemiological relationship between different strains on a farm or among different farms. The genotyping or characterisation method most used currently is genome sequencing, which nowadays is especially applied to PRRSV (figs. 15a and b).

Sample collection and submission

Sample collection is a critical point and caution should be taken to avoid cross-contamination or sample degradation. Samples to be tested by molecular techniques should be submitted as quickly as possible and kept chilled/frozen during transport. Special care should be taken when ISH for RNA sequences is required, since the activity of RNA-ases (which destroy RNA molecules) is increased when the animal is dead. However, fixation stops the activity of these enzymes. Therefore, the sooner the tissue is collected and preserved (fixed), the better.

Recommendations of use

The selection of the molecular technique to be used will depend on the type of pathogen (DNA or RNA).

Most of the abovementioned molecular methods are rapid, easy-to-perform and can be automated, enabling the analysis of

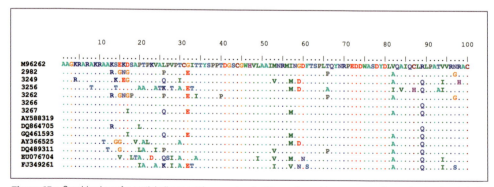

Figure 15a. Graphic view of a partial alignment (comparison) of the amino acid sequences of non-structural protein 2 (861 amino acids) for different PRRSV strains (listed in the left column). Each coloured letter represents a different amino acid in the protein sequence; the dots correspond to the amino acids that are in the same position as those in the first line.

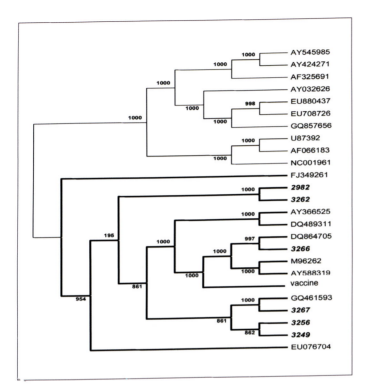

Figura 15b. Phylogenetic tree based on open reading frames (ORFs) 1 to 7 sequences of PRRSV isolates. Bootstrap values for each branch are shown as a number of coincident iterations over 1,000. The thick lines correspond to genotype I strains.

a high-throughput volume of samples. This is not the case of ISH. This latter technique requires tissue from dead animals and is more time-consuming. ISH is only used when the detection of the pathogen in the pathognomonic lesions is required, as in the case of PCV2.

The use of these molecular techniques is recommended in infectious diseases in which the mere presence of the pathogen implies disease development or has a direct impact on the animal's health or on the productive parameters, as in the cases of PRRS, ASF and CSF. On the other hand, the use of these techniques to establish a diagnosis in ubiquitous or widespread infections (e. g. for PCV2) is not recommended. Also, these techniques are useful to confirm the absence of the pathogen in eradication programmes (e. g. *Actinobacillus pleuropneumoniae* or *Mycoplasma hyopneumoniae*).

Caution should be taken when these techniques are used to detect highly genetically variable pathogens. All these laboratory methods are based on the ability of the specific primers or probes to match to the target DNA/RNA. Therefore, if the pathogen or DNA/RNA target is highly variable, false negative results can be obtained. In those cases, it is recommended to use molecular methods designed to detect conservative regions of the pathogen's genome or, alternatively, to run different tests using different pairs of primers or probes.

Results interpretation

In PCR, nPCR, RT-PCR or multiplex PCR procedures, the amplified genome is observed in agarose gel. The samples that yield a band in the gel are considered positive (fig. 16). In multiplex PCR, the different set of primers amplifies fragments of different lengths, yielding bands of different molecular weight (fig. 17).

No agarose gel is needed in qPCR techniques; qPCR machines are connected to a computer and a programme detects at which cycle of amplification fluorescence is first emitted. The earlier fluorescence is emitted, the higher the pathogen load is in the sample (fig. 18).

ISH is a colorimetric technique. Therefore, a sample will be positive (hybrids are present) when the nucleic acid is coloured (fig. 19).

All these techniques are based on the exponential amplification of a target DNA sequence (except ISH) and annealing of a specific DNA fragment to the diagnostic specimen. Therefore, caution should be taken with sample cross-contamination. To ensure good laboratory practices and the correct interpretation of the results, negative and positive controls should be included in each test.

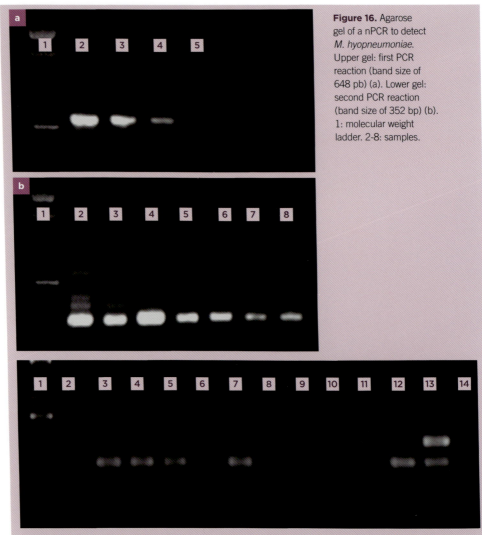

Figure 16. Agarose gel of a nPCR to detect *M. hyopneumoniae*. Upper gel: first PCR reaction (band size of 648 pb) (a). Lower gel: second PCR reaction (band size of 352 bp) (b). 1: molecular weight ladder. 2-8: samples.

Figure 17. Agarose gel of multiplex PCR to detect different virulent and non-virulent *Haemophilus parasuis* (Hp) strains. 1: molecular weight ladder; 2-5, 7 and 10: non-virulent Hp strains; 6: negative control; 8-9 and 11-14: virulent Hp strains.

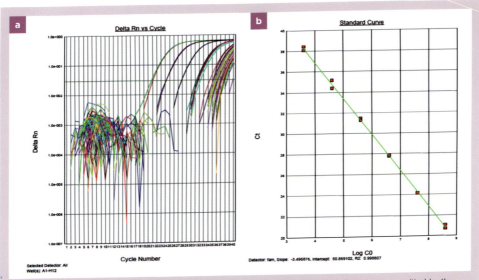

Figure 18. PCV2 qPCR amplification plot for several samples (a). Detection of the fluorescence emitted by the probe when PCV2 DNA is amplified. PCV2 Standard Curve (b). Cycle of detection of log10 dilutions of a plasmid with a known concentration of the target PCV2 sequence.

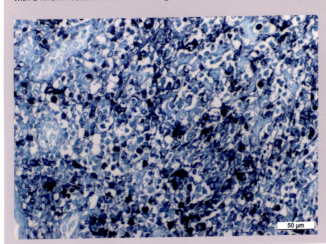

Figure 19. *In situ* hybridisation to detect PCV2, lymph node. Numerous macrophages and multinucleated giant cells stained in blue containing specific viral nucleic acid. Fast green counterstain.

SEROLOGICAL TECHNIQUES

Serology is the branch of laboratory medicine dealing with the detection of antibodies in blood serum in order to demonstrate an infection or a previous contact with a given antigen. In a broad sense, serology also includes antibody testing in other biological matrices such as oral fluids.

Reasons for serologic testing are varied and usually include the impossibility of reaching a definitive diagnosis just by examining the pigs, observing the gross lesions and considering the epidemiology of the process. Serological diagnosis is thus a complementary strategy to other diagnostic tests and an alternative when a microbiological diagnosis is not feasible or possible. Serological tests are generally cheap, rapid, sensitive and specific.

In addition to disease diagnosis, serologic testing may be required to identify the dynamics of a given infection in a herd, in what is called "serological profiling". Serology can also be applied to avoid the introduction of infected animals, for eradication purposes and to assess vaccine efficacy or monitor the response to a treatment. Moreover, export permits often require at least serological evidence of the absence of certain pathogens.

Basic concepts in serologic testing

Serologic testing is based on the capacity of detecting the presence of antibodies specific for a given pathogen. Therefore, the dynamics of the humoral response to the analysed pathogen determine the practical performance of a given test. The general scheme of the humoral response (fig. 20) indicates that, after encountering the antigen for the first time, there is an initial phase (days to weeks) during which the animal does not have any antibodies but is in the process of developing a humoral response. Then, antibodies of the IgM class appear and, after a few weeks, the IgG increases. In recall responses the IgG predominates. Thus, high levels of IgM are usually indicative of a very recent infection. On the contrary, if IgG is predominant, this means that the onset of the infection took place at least several weeks earlier. Similarly, paired testing of an individual at a two to three-week interval allows the determination of whether the antibody levels are increasing, decreasing or in a steady state. When a change from a negative to a positive status or a significant increase (usually 4-fold) is observed -what is called seroconversion-, this means that the animal has been infected recently or during the sampling interval.

Quantifying the amount of specific antibodies is therefore essential to the diagnosis. In the serology jargon, the term "titre" is used to refer to the amount of antibodies specific for a given antigen or, more precisely, the maximum dilution of the serum that reacts positively in an assay against a given pathogen.

Two other central concepts in serologic testing are sensitivity and specificity. Both concepts can be considered from either an analytical or a diagnostic point of view. Analytical sensitivity is the minimum amount of analyte (in this case, of specific antibodies) that a test can detect. Analytical specificity is the ability of a test to avoid the erroneous detection of partially cross-reactive antibodies. Diagnostic sensitivity is the performance of a test in the correct identification of infected animals as positive and depends on analytical sensitivity. Diagnostic specificity is the accuracy of an assay in the identification of non-infected pigs as negative (it depends on analytical specificity). False negative results (infected animals classified as negative by the test) and false positive results (healthy animals classified as positive) derive from a lack of diagnostic sensitivity and diagnostic specificity (fig. 21).

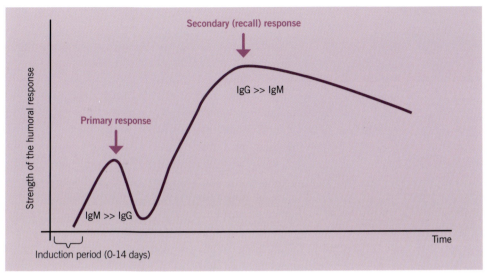

Figure 20. Development of the humoral (antibody) response. Initial response predominated by IgM. Over time (usually 2-4 weeks), the amount of IgM will decrease and IgG will increase. In subsequent contacts with the antigen a memory response develops.

Sampling in serologic testing

In swine medicine, herd or batch diagnosis is often as important as individual diagnosis. As a matter of fact, the usual approach to diagnose an outbreak of a disease -not to mention for its monitoring- is to sample a number of representative individuals (see chapter 2). Ensuring the quality and the representativeness of the samples is critical to take full advantage of the diagnostic power of serological techniques.

The quality of the serum sample is ensured by means of appropriate blood sample collection, submission and storage procedures. A convenient method for blood collection is the use of vacuum tubes. Blood samples should be allowed to clot for several hours at < 25 °C before centrifugation. Serum may be stored at 2-8 °C for up to 1 week or at ≤ -20 °C for longer storage times. No-frost freezers should be avoided. In general, whole blood or haemolysed sera are not acceptable for serological testing.

The approach to select the individuals to be tested is not the same in the case of an outbreak as for monitoring. In an outbreak, sampling is mostly directed to diseased individuals. In acute processes of short duration (for example, influenza), animals may not develop antibodies until a later phase, when the signs of the disease have disappeared and the determination of seroconversion is thus mandatory. Moreover, for common swine diseases, the inclusion of non-affected animals may provide valuable information. For the monitoring of diseases, sampling requires a statistical approach (see chapter 2). As a general rule, the sample size should provide a reasonable level of confidence (usually > 95%) that a low prevalence (for example 10%) will be detected. This ensures the early detection of the infection. Thirty samples ensure a prevalence of 10% and a 95% confidence level.

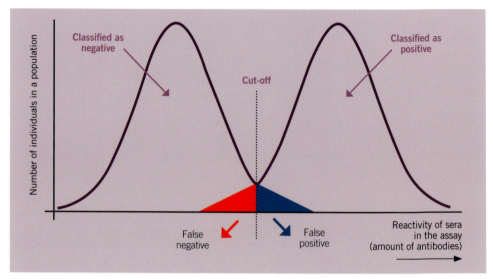

Figure 21. Diagnostic sensitivity and specificity are inherent properties of a diagnostic test that depend on the cut-off to distinguish between negative and positive individuals. The optimal cut-off is the one ensuring that the test produces a minimum proportion of false positive and negative results given the inherent characteristics of the test.

Most commonly used serological tests

Many different serological tests have been developed for the diagnosis of swine diseases, although in current laboratory practice the number of techniques used is very limited. This section reviews some of the techniques most commonly used.

ELISA: ELISA tests are the most popular assays for serological diagnosis nowadays. Technically, ELISA assays are based on the detection of specific antibodies by means of an "enzymatic conjugate", namely, an enzyme that reacts with an added substrate to produce a visible colour reaction.

The most common type of ELISA is indirect ELISA. In this test, an antigen is adsorbed to the wells of a plastic microtitre plate. Serum is added to the wells. If antibodies specific for the antigen are present in the serum, they will react with the antigen and remain attached to the plastic plate. In a subsequent step, an enzyme-conjugated antibody raised against pig IgG or IgM is added and, finally, a substrate for the enzyme is incorporated. If the serum contains specific antibodies, a colour reaction is observed; if not, the wells remain colourless. The results are read using a spectrophotometer. In indirect ELISA, the formation of colour in the wells is proportional to the amount of antibodies in the serum and to the number of enzyme-conjugated molecules bound. Therefore, this technique allows a semi-quantification of antibodies if a positive control sample with a known amount of antibodies is included. The spectrophotometric readings of the sample and the positive control can be used to calculate a ratio (S/P ratio) that indicates a relative "positivity".

A second type of ELISA commonly used in swine diagnosis is competitive ELISA. The main advantage of competitive ELISA is that it does not require species-specific conjugates; the disadvantage is that readouts are only in terms of positive/negative (fig. 22).

Haemagglutination inhibition: this assay is based on the ability of some antigens to agglutinate red blood cells and to induce antibodies inhibiting such capacity. It has an acceptable sensitivity and specificity and is useful to distinguish serotypes or serological variants, but is very cumbersome to perform and requires a constant source of red blood cells. Nowadays, its use is limited almost only to influenza and, occasionally, to porcine parvovirus (fig. 14).

Immunofluorescence antibody test: the principle of this test is based on an antigen-antibody reaction that takes place on a solid surface -usually a slide- where a particulate antigen or infected cells have been fixed. The reaction is revealed by the use of an anti-pig IgG antibody labelled with fluorescein (or other fluorophores). This technique allows titration and is highly specific if the reaction is read by a well-trained technician.

Complement fixation test: this assay is directed to detecting antibodies that have the ability to act together with a complement protein to produce the lysis of the pathogen. This assay was very popular to detect antibodies against various bacteria (e. g. *Brucella* spp.) and viruses. However, more modern techniques have almost made it obsolete.

Viral neutralisation test: the viral neutralisation test is aimed at detecting the presence in serum of antibodies that block the infectivity of a virus. The most common format requires the incubation of a dilution series of the serum samples with a fixed amount of the virus. Subsequently, the serum-virus mixture is added to target cells susceptible to the viral infection and the cell cultures are incubated in order to allow non-neutralised viruses to infect cells. The reaction is revealed by the observation of a specific cytopathic effect or,

more accurately, by using a fluorescent or enzyme-labelled antibody directed against the viral antigens. This test allows the titration of the serum and in most cases a direct interpretation of the "protection" given by the humoral response (although this is not always the case since in some viral infections such as PRRS, neutralising antibodies does not allow the prediction of the protection).

Agglutination tests: these tests are based on the binding of antibodies to particulate antigens that can agglutinate. The main advantage of agglutination assays is their sensitivity (they can detect early IgM responses) and for this reason they are valuable as screening tests; however, their lack of specificity requires confirmation of positive results by other tests. Agglutination tests are common for the diagnosis of *Brucella* spp.

Agar gel diffusion test and precipitation tests: these tests are mostly obsolete for the diagnosis of swine diseases.

Interpretation of results for some common pig diseases

The previous sections reviewed the basic aspects of serological diagnosis, which provide the grounds for a correct interpretation of results. However, apart from this, contextualisation is essential for an accurate interpretation of the results of serological tests. A first point to consider is that, in most cases, the serological tests currently sold for pigs do not allow the differentiation between vaccinated and infected pigs or between maternally-derived antibodies and actively-produced antibodies. A second point is the time required for antibodies to develop, which, in the case of pigs, can substantially differ depending on the pathogens. Thirdly, the use of different techniques for a given pathogen may produce different results. Table 3 summarises some critical aspects for the interpretation of serological results in pigs for some diseases.

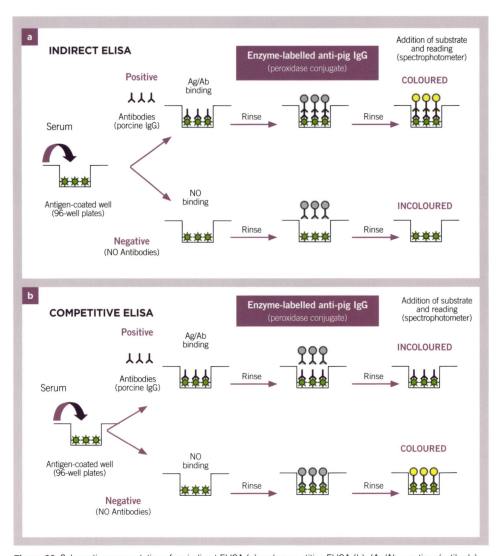

Figure 22. Schematic representation of an indirect ELISA (a) and competitive ELISA (b). (Ag/Ab = antigen/antibody). A positive indirect ELISA result in serum implies a change in colour, while there is no colour change in the negative serum. On the other hand, a change of colour in a competitive ELISA is interpreted as a negative result, while a slight or no colour change is observed in positive serum.

TABLE 3. Summary of the serological techniques most commonly used according to the pathogen and critical aspects for the interpretation of these tests.

Pathogen	Tests	Time to develop antibodies [a]	Duration of antibodies after infection	Fade out of maternally-derived antibodies	DIVA	Others
P. multocida toxin	ELISA	Up to 3 months	Months	6-8 weeks	No	Some infected pigs do not develop antibodies against the toxin.
A. pleuro-pneumoniae	ELISA, CFT	Approx. 7-14 days	Months	6-8 weeks	No	Serotype or serogroup specific.
M. hyopneu-moniae	ELISA	2-6 weeks	Months	6-8 weeks	No	Depending on the antigens used in the assay, cross-reactivity with *M. flocculare* may occur.
SIV	ELISA, HAI	Approx. 5-10 days	Weeks to months	6-8 weeks	No	ELISA tests are mostly directed to nucleocapsid proteins, HAI allows subtyping.
PRRSV	ELISA, IFA, VNT	Approx. 7-14 days for ELISA and IFA, several weeks for VNT	≤6-9 months	3-5 weeks	No	Some tests allow differentiation of genotype 1 and 2.
ADV/PRV	ELISA, cELISA, VNT	5-14 days	Years	10-14 weeks	Yes*	A single test is enough if DIVA vaccines are used.
B. suis	Agglutination test (Rose Bengal), CFT, ELISA	5-14 days	Months to years	Weeks	NA	None of the tests alone reach 95% sensitivity and specificity simultaneously. Combined testing is needed.
PCV2	ELISA	14-21 days	Months to years (?)	6-9 weeks	No	IgM and IgG testing available commercially.

Continued ▶

TABLE 3. (Continuation). Summary of the serological techniques most commonly used according to the pathogen and critical aspects for the interpretation of these tests.

Pathogen	Tests	Time to develop antibodies [a]	Duration of antibodies after infection	Fade out of maternally-derived antibodies	DIVA	Others
PPV	ELISA, HAI	5-14 days	Years	16-24 weeks	No	Vaccination titres tend to be lower than infection titres.
TGEV	cELISA	7-14 days	Years	≤8 weeks	NA	Cross-reactivity with porcine respiratory coronavirus.
L. intracellularis	ELISA, IFA	14-21 days	Months (?)	4-6 weeks (?)	No	Not used very often.
Salmonella spp.	ELISA	7-21 days	4 months	6-9 weeks	No	ELISA are serogroup specific.
E. rhusiopathiae	ELISA, microagglutination	10-14 days	Months to years (?)	≤8 weeks	No	Vaccination induces high levels of antibodies.
L. biflexa	Microagglutination	5-10 days	Months (?)	≤8 weeks (?)	NA	Available only in specialised laboratories.
SVDV	ELISA, VNT	5-14 days	Months to years (?)	≤8 weeks (?)	NA	VNT is the more specific test. Subject to legal regulations.
FMDV	ELISA, VNT	7-14 days	Years	8-10 weeks	No	Subject to legal regulations.
CSFV	cELISA, VNT	10-15 days	Years	8-10 weeks	Yes**	Subject to legal regulations.
ASFV	ELISA	5-8 days	Years	8-10 weeks	NA	Subject to legal regulations.

[a] In infection.

(?): limited data.

DIVA: Differentiating Infected from Vaccinated Animals.

NA: not applicable.

c-ELISA: competitive ELISA.

*If gE- vaccines are used.

** Only for vaccines licensed in the European Union for use in emergency case.

PARASITOLOGICAL METHODS

Coprological methods

Faeces for coprological analyses should be collected directly from the rectum of the animal. If this is not possible, samples should be collected immediately after defecation; otherwise, free-living soil nematodes and other pseudo-parasites rapidly invade the faecal sample.

Analyses should be conducted on fresh faecal material. For the presence of protozoan trophozoites, the samples should be examined immediately after collection, because these fragile organisms do not survive for long periods outside of the host. If the collected faeces cannot be examined within a few hours, the sample should be refrigerated. Helminth eggs and protozoan cysts are more resistant forms, but refrigeration does not stop their development and this can difficult their identification. Faeces should not be frozen, because freezing can distort parasite eggs.

Before performing any specific test, stools should be examined macroscopically to observe their consistency, colour and the presence of mucus, blood, adult parasites or tapeworm segments. Several coprological techniques can then be used to search for the presence of different parasitic forms:

Direct smear

The sensitivity of this method is very low and it is therefore not recommended for routine analysis. Nevertheless, it is sometimes used first to detect motile protozoan trophozoites. The technique consists in mixing, on a slide, a small amount of faeces with saline solution (concentrated solutions cannot be used as protozoan trophozoites are fragile). If the faecal layer is very thin, it may be possible to distinguish the movement of trophozoites. To observe internal structures, in some cases it is advisable to add a drop of Lugol's iodine stain to smears.

TABLE 4. Most common parasites diagnosed by coprological tests in pigs.

Parasite	Usual location/size	Cycle	Diagnostic/Infective stage
Ascaris suum (Large round worm)	▪ Small intestine, bile ducts, stomach ▪ 15-30 cm	Direct	Egg/embryonated egg (oral)
Strongyloides ramsoni (Threadworm)	▪ Small intestine of suckling pigs ▪ 3.3-4.5 mm	Direct	Egg/larvae (transplacental, transcolostral, oral, cutaneous)
Trichuris suis (Whipworm)	▪ Caecum and large intestine ▪ 5-8 cm	Direct	Egg/embryonated egg (oral)
Hyostrongylus rubidus (Red stomach worm)	▪ Stomach ▪ < 10 mm	Direct	Egg/larvae (oral)
Oesophagostomum spp. (Nodular worm)	▪ Caecum and colon ▪ 10-20 mm	Direct	Egg/larvae (oral)
Isospora suis/Eimeria spp. (Coccidia)	▪ Small intestine	Direct	Oocyst/sporulate oocyst (oral)
Balantidium coli	▪ Caecum and colon	Direct	Cyst/cyst (oral)

Qualitative flotation procedure

1. Mix about 2-3 g of faeces with a small amount of water and strain the mixture through a double layer of cheesecloth over a sieve into a centrifuge tube of 10 ml (fig. 23).
2. Put the tubes in a centrifuge at 650 G (approx. 1500-2000 rpm) for 5 minutes.
3. Discard the supernatant, re-suspend the sediment with the flotation solution (zinc o sucrose) and repeat the previous step.
4. Fill the tubes with additional flotation fluid until there is a reverse meniscus on the top. Place a cover slip and leave it to stand for at least 10 minutes; remove the cover slip, place it on a slide (fig. 24) and examine it with a microscope (observation with a 100x and 400x magnification).

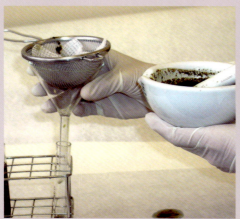
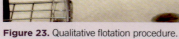

Figure 23. Qualitative flotation procedure.

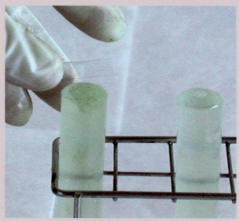

Figure 24. Qualitative flotation procedure.

Faecal flotation

This method is based on the principle that parasite eggs are less dense than the flotation medium, and thus float to the top of the tube or container. Different solutions can be used (saturated sodium chloride, saturated sodium nitrate, a 33% zinc sulphate solution or Sheather's sugar solution). A 33% zinc sulphate solution is prepared with 330 g of zinc sulphate, adding water to reach a volume of 1,000 ml. It is recommended to adjust the specific gravity (1.18) with a hydrometer. Sheather's solution (specific gravity 1.2-1.25) is prepared by mixing 454 g of sugar (sucrose) with 355 ml of hot water; to avoid contamination, 6 ml of formaldehyde are added when the solution is cooled at room temperature.

Faecal sedimentation

Sedimentation is used to isolate eggs of flukes and other tapeworms and nematodes whose eggs do no float readily in common flotation solutions. Sedimentation tests only have a limited concentrating ability and the sediment obtained contains many artefacts and dirt, and it is more difficult to detect the presence of parasites.

Quantitative flotation procedure (modified McMaster test)

1. Place 2 g of faeces in a ceramic mortar or in a beaker. Add 28 ml of zinc sulphate (specific gravity: 1.18). Homogenise the mixture completely.
2. Filter the sample into a beaker through a double layer of cheesecloth over a sieve, using a funnel. Press the cheesecloth to drain the liquid. Hold the filtrate under constant stirring using a magnetic stirrer.
3. Immediately fill the two chambers of a McMaster slide (0.15 ml each) using a Pasteur pipette and allow the slide to sit for 5-10 minutes (fig. 25).
4. Focus on the lines of the grid on the surface of the chamber using the 10x objective. Count the total number of eggs, oocysts and larvae. Each type of parasite should be counted separately.
5. Calculate the average counts of both chambers and multiply by 100. This result determines the number of parasite (oocysts, eggs, larvae, etc.) per gram.

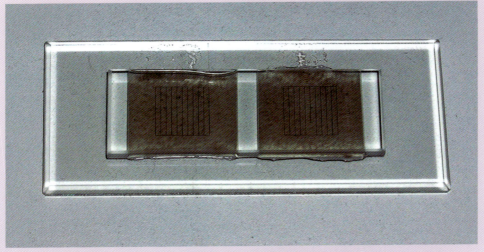

Figure 25. Quantitative flotation procedure. McMaster slide for faecal counts

Baermann technique

The Baermann technique is used to isolate larvae from faecal samples. In fresh samples it is used to diagnose lungworm infections (*Metastrongylus* spp.). This method also allows the detection of other nematodes in non-fresh samples, such as some parasitic larvae hatching from parasite eggs (*Strongyloides* spp., *Oesophagostomum* spp., *Hyostrongylus* spp.) and free-living nematodes from soil contamination. The sample is placed in a tea strainer and immersed in water in a sealed funnel (fig. 26). The nematode larvae, which are unable to swim against gravity, descend to the bottom of the funnel. A 10-hour wait approximately is required before the larvae are recovered.

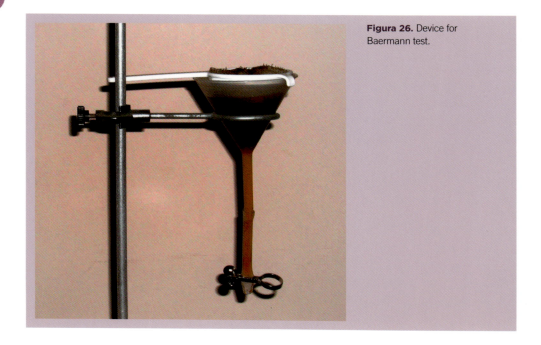

Figura 26. Device for Baermann test.

Methods for the diagnosis of sarcoptic mange

1. Scratching index (SI)

Pigs are observed for behaviour indicative of pruritus. Approximately 50 pigs are observed for 15 minutes. The SI is calculated by counting the total number of scratching episodes divided by the number of pigs observed. A threshold value of 0.4 can be used; values above or below are said to indicate the presence or absence of scabies.

2. Ear scrapings

The ear and external auditory canal are removed from the carcass at slaughter and the entire skin from the inside of the ear is scraped with a curette (fig. 27).

The scrapings can be examined under a stereo microscope for the presence of viable *S. scabiei* after exposure at 28 °C for 30 min (fig. 28). The examination of the negative scrapings using a digestion of the crusts with 10% potassium hydroxide, followed by a sedimentation–flotation technique, with sucrose is a recommended method (see chapter 10). The same technique can be performed in vivo, for example in sows.

3. Average dermatitis score (ADS)

The presence of erythematous papular dermatitis is determined for each carcass after scalding on a minimum of 50 animals. A score (0-3) is given according to the severity of the skin lesions (fig. 29). The ADS is calculated as the arithmetic mean of the individual scores. A threshold value for ADS of 0.5 is used as a reference to indicate the presence (> 0.5) or absence (< 0.5) of sarcoptic mange.

4. Serology

Serum samples can be examined for the presence of specific serum antibodies with an indirect ELISA technique. Free-living mite extracts, as a source of antigens, can give a specificity of 97% and a sensitivity of 78%.

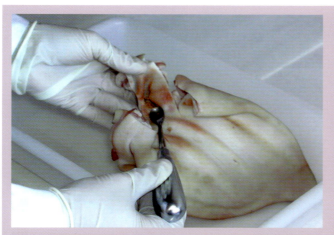

Figure 27. Ear scraping with curette.

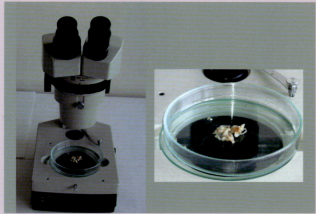

Figure 28. Scraping examined under a stereo microscope.

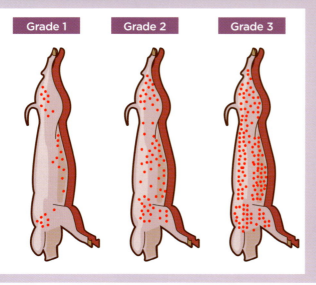

Grade 1   Grade 2   Grade 3

Figure 29. Papular dermatitis scoring at slaughter (From National Animal Disease Information Service; http://www.nadis.org.uk).

5

Laboratory diagnosis of respiratory disorders

INTRODUCTION

Disorders and diseases involving the respiratory system are probably the most frequent disease problems in swine production. The vast majority of swine respiratory disorders are caused by infectious agents, but environmental factors and management practices (e. g. temperature, ventilation, pig density and production system) together with the immune status of the pig play a fundamental predisposing role. The negative impact of some infectious agents (mainly viruses) and environmental factors on the mucociliary barrier of the airways and the phagocytic capacity of macrophages facilitate the invasion of the lung tissue by bacteria that colonise the upper respiratory tract. Some infectious agents (such as *Actinobacillus pleuropneumoniae*) are primary respiratory pathogens and are less influenced by predisposing factors.

Respiratory diseases are usually observed as herd outbreaks, with variable morbidity and mortality rates. They can range from mild disease signs with a reduced feed intake, to severe respiratory diseases with a high mortality rate. Primary infectious agents may cause diseases and lesions alone, but several pathogens are usually involved in respiratory diseases. This fact, and the impossibility to distinguish the different infectious agents involved on the basis of clinical signs alone, has led to the use of the term porcine

TABLE 1. Main infectious and non-infectious causes of respiratory disorders in pigs.

Agent (disease)	Disorder/Clinical signs
PRCV	Subclinical, ubiquitous.
Porcine cytomegalovirus (inclusion body rhinitis)	Subclinical or mild rhinitis, ubiquitous.
Toxigenic *P. multocida* (progressive atrophic rhinitis)	Atrophy and loss of turbinates, deviation of snout, reduced growth.
Toxigenic *B. bronchiseptica* (regressive atrophic rhinitis)	Atrophy and loss of turbinates, deviation of snout.
M. hyopneumoniae (enzootic pneumonia)	Productive cough, reduced feed intake.
A. pleuropneumoniae (porcine pleuropneumonia)	Productive cough, fever, variable mortality rate.
P. multocida (pneumonic pasteurellosis)	Productive cough, fever.
A. suis	Sudden death, dyspnoea, cutaneous signs.
PRRSV (PRRS)	Hacking cough, dyspnoea, growth retardation, subcutaneous lymphadenopathy.
PCV2 (PCV2-SD)	Hacking cough, dyspnoea, growth retardation, subcutaneous lymphadenopathy.
SIV (swine influenza)	Cough, fever; often subclinical.
Ammonia and dust	Sneezing and cough, predisposing factor for bacterial pneumonia.
Metastrongylus spp.	Cough.
A. suum	Dyspnoea (*larva migrans*).

respiratory disease complex (PRDC) to refer to respiratory diseases of multifactorial origin in growing/finishing pigs. The agents most commonly involved in PRDC are PRRSV, PCV2, SIV and *Mycoplasma hyopneumoniae*. These agents may predispose to secondary bacterial pneumonia, or even to systemic bacterial infections (*Haemophilus parasuis* polyserositis). Table 1 shows the main infectious and non-infectious causes of respiratory disorders in pigs.

Herd factors significantly influence the manifestations of respiratory diseases. Therefore, when facing respiratory problems, it is essential to take action regarding the issues raised in table 2.

CLINICAL EXAMINATION

The morbidity and mortality rates associated to respiratory diseases may vary considerably depending on the herd immunity to the different pathogens, management factors and stressors. Clinical signs may include dyspnoea (laboured breathing), tachypnoea (rapid breathing), cough and nasal and ocular discharge. Fever, anorexia, cyanosis, and sudden death may occur in cases of severe disease, such as those caused by *A. pleuropneumoniae*. Some viral agents, such as PRCV, cause subclinical infections, and others such as SIV cause a subclinical or mild disease, eventually associated with growth retardation and a reduced feed conversion ratio. On the other hand, infections by PRRSV and/or PCV2 (causing PCV2-SD) may lead to severe respiratory signs (dyspnoea, tachypnoea) but also to a systemic disease with a variety of signs that are not limited to the respiratory system. The aetiological clarification of PRDC episodes requires a necropsy and laboratory investigation.

TABLE 2. Herd factors with a significant influence on the outcome of respiratory diseases.

Generic factors	Specific factors
Production system	▪ Large herd size. ▪ High stocking density. ▪ Continuous flow. ▪ Introduction of pigs from different sources or from herds with an unknown or low sanitary status.
Housing	▪ Bad insulation and ventilation. ▪ Open partitions between pens. ▪ Large rooms. ▪ Slatted floors.
Nutrition	▪ Insufficient caloric intake. ▪ Insufficient amount of macro- and micronutrients in feed.
Management	▪ Poor monitoring of disease signs. ▪ Incorrect vaccination plans and other preventive measures. ▪ Poor caretaking of diseased pigs. ▪ Poor hygiene. ▪ Poor biosecurity. ▪ Excess of cross-fostering.

PATHOLOGICAL ASSESSMENT

Rhinitis and tracheitis

Inflammation of the nasal mucosa or rhinitis is a frequent sign of some diseases of the upper respiratory tract. It is manifested by sneezing and by a serous to muco-purulent nasal exudate. Bacteria such as *Bordetella bronchiseptica* and *Pasteurella multocida* and viruses such as porcine cytomegalovirus are the main causes of catarrhal to muco-purulent rhinitis in pigs. However, toxigenic *B. bronchiseptica* and *P. multocida* are the infectious agents of regressive (RAR) and progressive (PAR) atrophic rhinitis, respectively. The main difference between them is that PAR is a systemic problem while RAR is just a local nasal disorder. Mucosal damage caused by irritation due to dust or ammonia can also lead to rhinitis.

Pneumonia

Grossly, pneumonia in pigs can be divided into four general types: suppurative bronchopneumonia, fibrinous necrotising pleuropneumonia, interstitial/broncho-interstitial pneumonia, and embolic pneumonia. The infectious agents are usually associated with one of these forms of pneumonia, and a correct morphological diagnosis can help to make hypotheses about the aetiological causes and decide on further diagnostic laboratory tests.

In **suppurative bronchopneumonia**, part of or the whole cranial and middle lobes are bilaterally consolidated and of a grey-pink colour. Suppurative exudation may be seen in the lumen of the bronchi on the cut surface. The pleural surface is not affected, and has a smooth and moist texture. This lesion is usually found in enzootic pneumonia (*M. hyopneumoniae*, although in most cases there is a co-infection with other bacteria such as *P. multocida*, *B. bronchiseptica*,

Streptococcus suis, etc.). In uncomplicated cases of enzootic pneumonia, the lesion may resolve totally. The affected areas are filled with exudate and sink in fluids such as formalin. Moreover, the previously mentioned bacteria can also cause suppurative pneumonia in the absence of *M. hyopneumoniae*, and they are usually secondary contributors to other damage in the lung mostly caused by viruses.

Fibrinous-necrotising pleuropneumonia is the result of an inflammatory process with a more severe alteration of vessel permeability, leading to the exudation of large plasma proteins, such as fibrinogen, which form fibrin clots within the alveoli. The fibrinous exudate makes the lung firm and the affected areas do not collapse when opening the chest. The pleurae are often affected by fibrinous exudation, with a thin layer of white-yellowish fibrin covering the affected areas of the lung. The interlobular septa and vessels are also filled with fibrin and distended, giving the cut surface a marble appearance. The large affected areas may undergo necrosis and have a haemorrhagic appearance. The affected areas are filled with exudates and sink in fluids such as formalin. In pigs, the agent most frequently associated with fibrinous-necrotising pleuropneumonia is *A. pleuropneumoniae*, but *P. multocida* may also cause a necrotising lesion (usually not haemorrhagic) in some cases. *Actinobacillus suis* has also been considered as the cause of a type of fibrinous-necrotising pneumonia that is very similar to that caused by *A. pleuropneumoniae*. The distribution of the lesions is wider than in suppurative bronchopneumonia and these mainly affect the cranio-ventral parts of the lung, although in the case of porcine pleuropneumonia, other portions of the lung may be affected (caudal lobes). The necrotising lesions do not resolve and may remain in the lung as sequestration or evolve as scars, with or without a fibrous adhesive pleuritis.

Interstitial pneumonia is a lesion that affects the lung in a diffuse manner, and originates from the haematogenous spread of viral agents to the lung tissue. The alveolar septa are enlarged, with an infiltration of lymphocytes, plasma cells and macrophages in the interstitial space. The alveoli also become filled with macrophages and the epithelial cells lining the alveolar walls (pneumocytes) may proliferate. The lungs do not collapse when opening the thoracic cavity and have a rubbery consistency. Interstitial pneumonia is usually caused by viruses, being PRRSV and PCV2, alone or in mixed infections, the most frequent causes.

SIV is responsible for **broncho-interstitial pneumonia**, which causes the lungs to have a lobular pattern and mainly affects the apical and middle lobes as well as, to a lesser extent, the diaphragmatic lobes. This distribution is consistent with the aerogenous spread of the virus within the lung. The original lesion caused by *M. hyopneumoniae* is also a broncho-interstitial pneumonia.

Embolic pneumonia is caused by the haematogenous dissemination of bacteria from other distant sites in the body, causing abscesses or necrotic lesions randomly distributed throughout the lung parenchyma. Septicaemic infections by *A. suis* cause necrotic foci in the pulmonary tissue, but these foci may be rather small and difficult to observe grossly.

Pleuritis

Pleuritis is the inflammation of the pleural surfaces. Fibrinous pleuritis is commonly found in infections caused by *H. parasuis*, *S. suis*, and *Mycoplasma hyorhinis*, usually as a part of a wider serosal involvement (polyserositis), polyarthritis and meningitis. The resorption of fibrin takes place due to its reorganisation with the connective tissue newly formed from the pleural surfaces, ending with the fibrous

adherence of the parietal and visceral serosal surfaces of the pleura (fibrous adhesive pleuritis), a very common finding at slaughter. The laboratory analysis of these chronic lesions is usually unsuccessful.

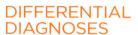

DIFFERENTIAL DIAGNOSES

The differential diagnosis of respiratory disorders is based on clinical signs, gross lesions and results of the laboratory investigation. The clinical signs are usually non-specific, and the clinical diagnosis may only be tentative. An accurate morphological classification of the lesions is of great relevance to direct the subsequent laboratory investigations.

Subclinical viral infections of the respiratory tract are prevalent. PRCV, a spike gene deletion mutant of TGEV (transmissible gastroenteritis virus), is ubiquitous in pig farms and usually circulates without causing any apparent symptoms. This virus may cause broncho-interstitial pneumonia, but this disease is rarely reported in practice; its importance in the context of PRDC is not well defined. The beneficial effect of a PRCV infection is that it gives protection against TGEV. Other viruses such as PCV2 and PRRSV can also cause subclinical infections, but these are generally systemic rather than exclusively respiratory. The diagnosis of these subclinical infections is mainly achieved by means of serological analyses (evidence of seroconversion) or detection of the virus in biological samples (lung or nasal cavity, or serum in case of systemic viral infections).

Sneezing and **nasal discharge** are frequent clinical signs observed in **atrophic rhinitis**. Lesions may develop at any age, but the pigs affected within the first few weeks of life show a more severe atrophic damage. The main lesion is a progressive atrophy of the ventral and dorsal turbinates, often accompanied by snout deviation. These alterations may be accompanied or not by mucopurulent rhinitis. The diagnosis in an individual animal is best done at necropsy or at slaughter, by a transversal section of the snout between the first and second lower premolar. Serological techniques (ELISA to detect antibodies to the *P. multocida* toxins) or PCR to detect the toxin gene are suitable for large scale diagnoses in living animals. **Sneezing** is the main clinical sign associated with inclusion body rhinitis (porcine cytomegalovirus infection). This virus causes a mild or subclinical infection in young piglets and affects the nasal mucosa, although it may become a systemic disease in immunosuppressed pigs. Many piglets are usually infected, but death seldom occurs. Macroscopically, serous or mucopurulent rhinitis may be present, but the final diagnosis has to be confirmed by histopathological examination, with the observation of characteristic, large round nuclear basophilic inclusion bodies distending the nuclei of the glandular and lining epithelial cells.

High fever, apathy, anorexia, cyanosis, tachycardia and tachypnea are the usual signs of peracute *A. pleuropneumoniae* infections. The affected pigs may die due to acute circulatory failure, lung oedema and necrosis. In acute cases there is a fever, dyspnoea, a deep productive cough and apathy, and pigs develop a severe fibrinous-necrotising pleuropneumonia. Chronic forms develop after clinical signs disappear. The affected animals survive with chronic respiratory lesions in the form of necrotic lung areas with fibrous demarcation (sequestration) and focal fibrous pleural adhesions. Acute forms are easy to diagnose by analysing their clinical and pathological features, but the detection of the bacteria by means of a standard isolation or PCR is confirmatory. Chronic forms are mainly suspected because the previously mentioned lesions are observed at slaughter checks; the

detection of the bacteria from chronic lesions is seldom successful.

Cough, fever, and dyspnoea are often observed, especially in growing and finishing pigs. The clinical distinction of respiratory diseases caused by specific agents or by combinations of them is not possible based only on clinical signs and pathological findings. Enzootic pneumonia (multifactorial, non-viral disease in which *M. hyopneumoniae* is the primary agent), alone or in a co-infection with viruses (SIV, PRRSV, PC2, etc. -and therefore the whole picture named PRDC-), needs a laboratory diagnostic clarification. The most commonly used analyses include serological follow-ups (cross-sectional antibody profiles or evidence of sero-conversion) or direct detection of the pathogen in biological samples including serum (systemic pathogens) and/or nasal swabs and lung (strict respiratory pathogens). More information on PRRSV and PCV2-SD can be found in chapter 7 (systemic diseases). Apart from their presentation as part of the PRDC, SIV infections may manifest with the typical presentation of an acute outbreak of coughing and fever. The individual diagnosis of SIV is established by the detection of SIV genome by means of RT-PCR in lung or lung secretions, and/or by the detection of microscopic lesions of bronchiolitis and of SIV antigen associated with these lesions in the epithelium of the airways.

The **sudden death** of young piglets may have several possible aetiologies, including bacterial septicaemias. *A. suis* is an opportunistic pathogen that may cause a septicaemic disease in pigs at any age. Multifocal, microscopic necrotising embolic lung involvement is common, together with haemorrhages and occasional fibrin in serosal surfaces (serofibrinous pleuritis) and other organs. Other systemic bacterial pathogens, such as *H. parasuis*, *S. suis* and rarely *Escherichia coli*, can also cause acute septicaemia leading to the death of the affected pigs in a few hours. These latter pathogens together with *M. hyorhinis* can also cause respiratory problems and growth retardation as part of a systemic picture of fibrinous polyserositis. The isolation of the bacteria from systemic sites confirms the diagnosis.

Cough with (usually) minimal concurrent clinical signs, and distributed quite randomly in a batch of pigs, be related to parasitic infestations. Adults of *Metastrongylus* spp. parasitise the airways of pigs and cause mucopurulent tracheobronchitis, which occludes the airways to a great extent and predisposes to bacterial infections. Diagnosis is established by observation of adult parasites (size of 40-50 mm) in bronchi, but a flotation test can be used (although eggs do not float well). The migration of larvae of *Ascaris suum* through the lung causes petechial bleeding and interstitial pneumonia. The presence of larvae in the lung may be demonstrated microscopically; moreover, flotation tests can be carried out at the laboratory.

A diagnostic algorithm of the main respiratory disorders based on clinical signs, lesions and laboratory techniques is presented in figure 1.

CLINICAL CASE

Clinical history

3-site farm with 7,000 sows. A respiratory disorder was observed in piglets at the end of the lactation and early nursery periods. The farm was seronegative against ADV and seropositive (stable) to PRRSV and *M. hyopneumoniae*. Production records were considered good, with acceptable mortality rates at the different production phases (14% during lactation, 2% in nursery pigs and 4% in fattening pigs). Piglets showed coughing, dyspnoea and a progressive loss of weight. The mortality rates increased from 14% to 18%

during lactation, and from 2% to 4% in nursery pigs. An infectious process was suspected and some animals were sent for necropsy and detailed laboratory investigation.

Pathological analysis

Four 3-week old pigs and three 4-week old pigs were submitted for necropsy. Macroscopically, their lungs showed a grey-pink cranio-ventral consolidation affecting large areas of the lung parenchyma, which was not collapsed (figs. 2 and 3). When the lungs were sectioned, a muco-purulent secretion exuded from the bronchi. Infections by PRRSV/SIV/PCV2 were suspected, with the potential participation of *M. hyopneumoniae* and a complicating secondary bacterial infection caused by infectious agents such as *B. bronchiseptica* or *P. multocida*.

Laboratory results

Histologically, there was a prominent purulent exudate in the alveoli and airways and damage of the bronchial epithelial layer (necrotising bronchiolitis). The RT-PCR results for PRRSV in lung samples and serum were negative. A PCR test for *M. hyopneumoniae* in lung samples also yielded a negative result. Therefore, the participation of these two agents was excluded at first. Inmunohistochemical (IHC) staining was performed on histological sections for PRRSV and SIV. The results were only positive for SIV in 2 out of 7 pigs (fig. 4). Laboratory studies for PCV2 (ISH) yielded negative results. No bacteriological studies, apart from that carried out for *M. hyopneumoniae*, were performed in these animals.

Discussion

Based on the clinical signs and lesions, a pneumonia caused by viruses with the possible participation of *M. hyopneumoniae* and a secondary bacterial complication was the preliminary diagnosis established after

FIGURE 1. Main differential diagnoses of general respiratory disorders in pigs.

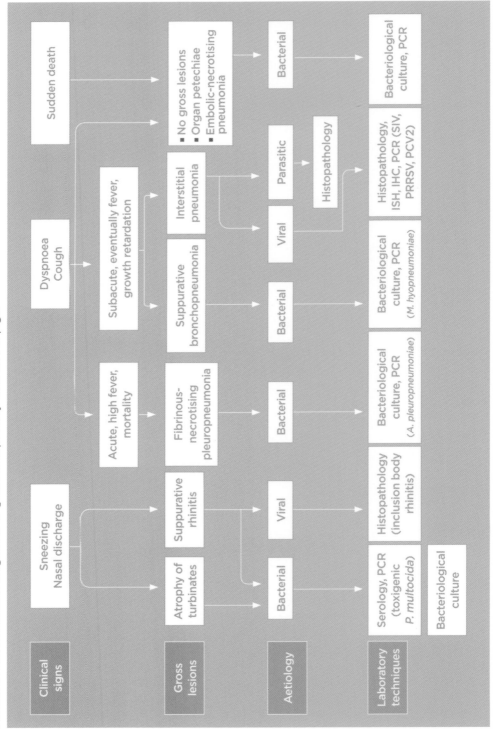

necropsy. It is true that the animals were very young to consider an enzootic pneumonia, but it certainly should be part of the differential diagnosis list. The laboratory results showed the participation of SIV in the process and the absence of PRRSV, PCV2 and *M. hyopneumoniae*. The global interpretation of the case was an infection by SIV with a complicating bacterial infection. The SIV was found by IHC in only 2 out of the 7 necropsied pigs, probably due to the short duration of the SIV infection. In a very large farm like the studied one (7,000 sows), it is difficult to control viral infections since it is usually possible to find subpopulations of pigs with different immunities. Vaccination against SIV was not attempted. The disease slowly evolved to a subclinical form in 6-8 months, when it was considered resolved spontaneously from a disease (not infection) point of view.

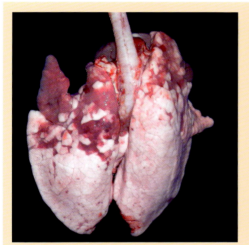

Figure 2. Lung, 3 week-old piglet. Moderate to marked pulmonary cranio-ventral consolidation with multifocal distribution in the apical and middle lobes, as well as in the cranial part of the left diaphragmatic lobe. These lesions are very suggestive of a broncho-interstitial pneumonia, which may be the result of SIV and/or *M. hyopneumoniae* infections.

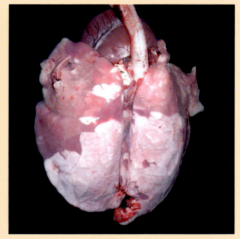

Figure 3. Lung, 4 week-old piglet. Marked and extensive pulmonary cranio-ventral consolidation, suggesting a catarrhal-purulent bronchopneumonia. This type of lesion indicates a bacterial participation.

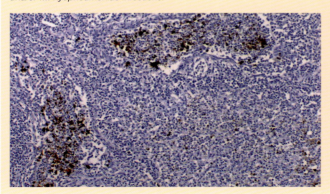

Figure 4. Lung, IHC to detect SIV. High amount of SIV antigen (brown staining) in the epithelial cells of the bronchioli as well as in the alveolar macrophages within the inflammatory infiltrates of the lung parenchyma.

6

Laboratory diagnosis of **enteric disorders**

INTRODUCTION

Enteric diseases are among the main causes of losses on swine operations. The importance of these processes derives not only from the mortality associated with outbreaks but also from the costs resulting from a decreased feed conversion efficiency, increased days to market and increased antibiotic usage. This chapter deals with enteric conditions as the primary manifestation of a disease; thus, systemic diseases or other diseases that can also cause diarrhoea or other enteric disorders are addressed in other chapters.

The most common enteric diseases in swine are of infectious origin and display an age-related distribution that reflects the epidemiology of each pathogen on the farm (fig. 1). In suckling pigs, the development of an enteric infectious disease is the result of a combination of factors that include the intrinsic characteristics of the newborn pig (e. g. lack of maternally-transferred antibodies), the immunity of the sow and the amount of colostrum and milk IgA ingested by the piglet, the circulation of specific pathogens (viruses, bacteria and parasites) as well as environmental conditions, particularly temperature and hygiene. In weaners, enteric diseases usually appear as soon as the maternally-derived IgA fades out (more precisely 1-2 weeks after weaning). The commingling of pigs from different litters –and therefore with different immune and health statuses– also contributes to the diffusion of pathogens. In fatteners and finishers, enteric diseases are often related to endemic pathogens and tend to manifest after mixing pigs in fattening units. In sows or boars, enteric diseases are not common unless a new pathogen is introduced on the farm. Dietary causes (e. g. hypersensitivity to soy meal) can also cause enteric conditions, although this rarely occurs. Finally, although

toxic substances may occasionally be found as causes of enteric diseases, this is not common.

CLINICO-PATHOLOGICAL EXAMINATION AND EPIDEMIOLOGY OF ENTERIC DISEASES IN PIGS

The most common manifestation of enteric diseases is diarrhoea, namely an increase in both the water content of faecal material and stool frequency. In practical situations, the watery consistency of the faeces and occasionally a change in their normal colour may be the only visible signs. The presence of mucus, fresh or digested blood or undigested feed is of importance in order to establish a differential diagnosis. Vomiting is another sign that may be observed in enteric processes, particularly in infections caused by enteric viruses. Rectal temperature is not always elevated even when infectious agents are the cause of the disorder and, thus, the detection of fever is a valuable finding; however, a normal rectal temperature does not exclude most enteric agents. In fact, some agonic animals may be hypothermic.

A necropsy can provide useful information for the orientation of the diagnosis, although in many instances it is difficult to reach a definitive diagnosis based solely on the necropsy findings. The predominant type of enteritis (catarrhal, ulcerative, necrotic, etc.) and the localisation of the lesions (small or large bowel, disseminated) are usually enough to reduce the number of potential causes involved in a differential diagnosis. However, the rapid autolysis of the gut after death (figs. 2a and b) requires a careful selection of the animals to be necropsied in order to collect valuable information.

The epidemiology of the disease provides valuable information. In suckling pigs, taking

FIGURE 1. Distribution of the causes of enteric diseases in pigs based on the age at which they are most commonly found. The dotted lines indicate that the process is only seen at those ages during epidemic episodes.

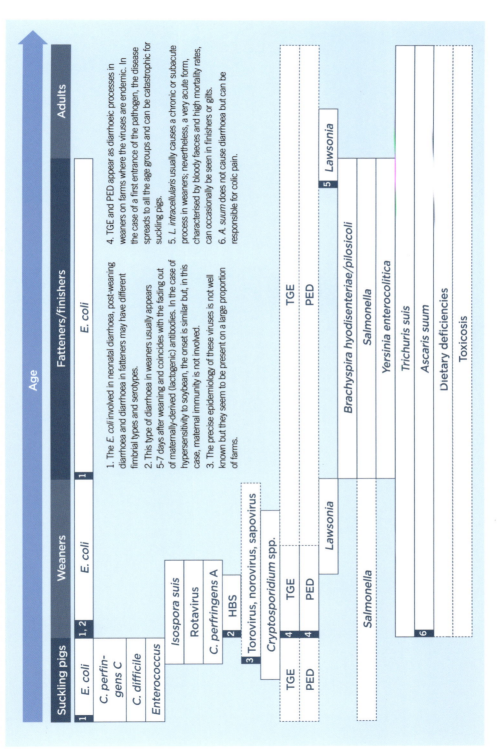

1. The *E. coli* involved in neonatal diarrhoea, post-weaning diarrhoea and diarrhoea in fatteners may have different fimbrial types and serotypes.

2. This type of diarrhoea in weaners usually appears 5–7 days after weaning and coincides with the fading out of maternally-derived (lactogenic) antibodies. In the case of hypersensitivity to soybean, the onset is similar but, in this case, maternal immunity is not involved.

3. The precise epidemiology of these viruses is not well known but they seem to be present on a large proportion of farms.

4. TGE and PED appear as diarrhoeic processes in weaners on farms where the viruses are endemic. In the case of a first entrance of the pathogen, the disease spreads to all the age groups and can be catastrophic for suckling pigs.

5. *L. intracellularis* usually causes a chronic or subacute process in weaners; nevertheless, a very acute form, characterised by bloody faeces and high mortality rates, can occasionally be seen in finishers or gilts.

6. *A. suum* does not cause diarrhoea but can be responsible for colic pain.

note of the number of affected litters, the proportion of affected piglets per litter and of the parity of the sows whose litters are affected may help to find the reasons behind an outbreak of diarrhoea. Usually, the diarrhoeic disorders in newborns caused by endemic agents (e. g. enteropathogenic *Escherichia coli*) and favoured by a poor adaptation of the sows tend to be concentrated in litters of first-parity sows, while the introduction of a new agent (e. g. transmissible gastroenteritis coronavirus) results in a generalised outbreak. The accumulation of cases of diarrhoea in a single animal in each litter, regardless of the parity of the sow, is an indication of a deficient intake of milk or of an increased number of weak-born piglets.

DIFFERENTIAL DIAGNOSES

In a very broad sense, the laboratory diagnosis of enteric diseases in pigs includes histopathological, microbiological, parasitological, serological and, eventually, toxicological analyses. The main limitation of the diagnosis is the quality of the samples due to the rapid autolysis of the intestinal tissue. As a general rule, the best samples are obtained from acutely affected animals and the best approach is to select one or more of them that will be euthanised and necropsied. Obviously, this is not always possible. If samples are to be taken from a pig found dead, it is important to remember that tissues obtained more than

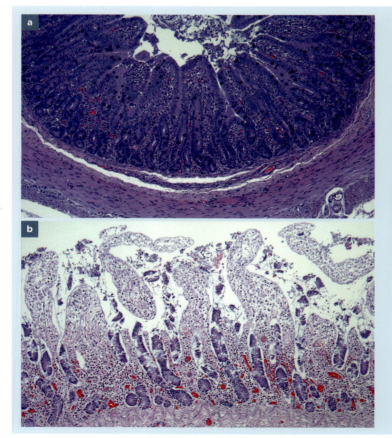

Figure 2. Histological picture of a fresh and well-preserved small intestine; the integrity of the microvilli and crypts allows the diagnosis of subtle alterations in the intestinal mucosa (a). Histological view of an autolytic small intestine; the marked loss of structure does not allow a proper pathological diagnosis. Post-mortem damage of the intestine implies changes in the population of bacteria, compromising a potential bacteriological diagnosis (b).

4-6 h after the death of the animal are not suitable for histopathological analyses. A similar criterion is applicable for microbiological analyses, although for some pathogens (e. g. enteropathogenic *E. coli*) detection is possible much later. In any case, it is always advisable to send both fresh and formalin-fixed samples to the laboratory since this allows a complete diagnosis. A decision chart for the collection of samples in an enteric disorder scenario is shown in figure 3. An explanation of how to collect and submit intestinal samples to the laboratory is given in chapters 2 and 3.

In general, the definitive diagnosis of an enteric problem will most often require the combination of several diagnostic techniques. A necropsy and histopathogical examination of the intestines (small and large) usually allow the identification or ruling out of the type of agent involved in the disorder, although they seldom allow the identification of a precise agent without further testing. For example, for most enteric viruses in pigs, diarrhoea is caused by their replication in mature enterocytes in the mid and upper part of the villi of the small intestine. As a result, there is a shortening of the villi. Other pathogens as *Brachyspira* spp. penetrate in the colonic mucosa and cause severe inflammation and eventually haemorrhages. Table 1 shows a summary of the lesions commonly seen in different enteric disorders in pigs.

Nowadays, classical bacteriological techniques are not sufficient for the identification of many enteric bacterial pathogens. Some of them are either non-culturable in conventional bacteriological media (e. g. *Lawsonia intracellularis*) or the culture has a low sensitivity (e. g. *Brachyspira* spp.). For other easily culturable bacteria such as *E. coli* or clostridia, the identification the virulence genes of the bacteria is crucial to ascertain their role in the clinical problem observed and to decide what vaccine should be selected for sows in the

case of neonatal diarrhoea. Thus, for *E. coli*, it is advisable to have some information on the type of fimbriae they possess and the enterotoxins they produce, as well as to determine if the strain harbours the intimin and EAST genes, which are important for attaching and effacing *E. coli*. For *Clostridium perfringens*, the determination of the presence of the different clostridial toxins by PCR is also helpful.

Regarding virology, in practical terms, classical virological isolation from faeces is seldom used as a diagnostic method. Alternative strategies such as the capture ELISA technique (rotavirus and coronavirus) or PCR are preferred because of their convenience. Techniques such as fluorescence labelling in frozen tissues are being less and less used. For parasites, coprological analyses (sedimentation/flotation, see chapter 4) are still the first choice techniques.

Serology is of little use in the diagnosis of most enteric outbreaks caused by nfectious and parasitic agents. Firstly, because of the lack of adequate serological tests and secondly, because in most cases, acutely affected pigs are still seronegative. Commercial serological tests for TGEV are available, but their usefulness is limited due to the cross-reactivity between this virus and PRCV, and because in very acute enteric infections the diseased animals are still seronegative. Table 2 summarises the tests most commonly used for the diagnosis of enteric conditions in pigs.

CLINICAL CASE

Clinical history

In its last 3 consecutive batches, a weaning unit of 600 piglets had suffered a problem of diarrhoea affecting weaners of six weeks of age onwards. The problem affected about 5%-10% of the piglets and the most evident sign was the loose consistency of the faeces, with the presence of undigested feed particles.

FIGURE 3. Flow chart for sampling for enteric diseases in pigs.

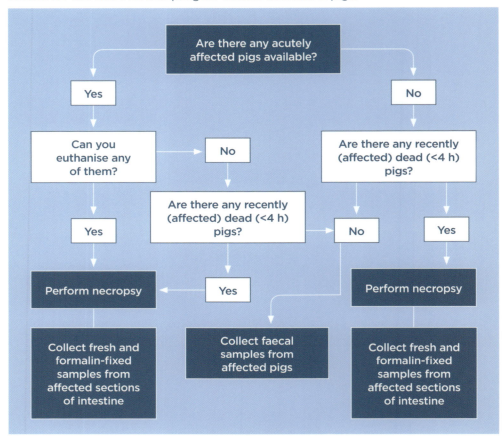

Some pigs showed a moderately distended abdomen. The problem persisted for the rest of the weaning phase and continued at the beginning of the fattening phase, which took place in a different location. The feed intake was normal and the mortality rate did not increase significantly compared to the historical records of the previous 12 months (1.0% *vs.* 1.5%). However, the average weight at the end of the weaning phase was lower than before the onset of the problem. The feed conversion ratio increased. This weaning unit received a batch of 3-week-old animals of a single origin every two weeks. The animals could come from two different sources, both PRRSV-free.

All the piglets were vaccinated against PCV2 on their arrival at the unit and, if needed, received medicated (colistin) feed during the first week at the nursery. The usual problems of this weaning unit were post-weaning diarrhoea that occurred about 1-2 weeks after entrance (usually diagnosed as colibacillosis) and, from time to time, some cases of oedema disease appeared (this was not the case at the time of the described disorder). Respiratory diseases were not a significant problem.

Differential diagnosis

Given the non-specificity of the signs described, several causes could lie behind the

TABLE 1. Summary of hallmark lesions in most common enteric diseases in swine.

Cause	Predominant localisation	Main (gross/microscopic) findings
Enterotoxigenic *E. coli* (ETEC)	Small intestine	Catarrhal enteritis, milk in the stomach, no (or slight) villous atrophy.
Attaching and effacing *E. coli* (AEEC)	Small and large intestine	Moderate to severe villous atrophy.
C. perfringens type C	Small intestine (jejunum)	Necrotising-haemorrhagic enteritis, intestinal emphysema.
C. perfringens type A	Small intestine (occasionally large)	Mild necrotising enteritis.
C. difficile	Large bowel	Mesocolonic oedema, multifocal erosive colitis.
L. intracellularis	Ileum (ileocecal valve)	Thickening (hyperplasic-proliferative enteritis) of the gut wall, necrotic enteritis. Haemorrhagic enteritis in the acute form.
B. hyodysenteriae	Colon (and occasionally cecum)	Erosive, ulcerative, haemorrhagic and/or necrotising enteritis
B. pilosicoli	Colon (and occasionally cecum)	Hyperaemia, oedematous surface, catarrhal enteritis.
Salmonella spp.	Large intestine	Catarrhal to fibrinous-necrotising enteritis, colitis and/or typhlitis.
Y. enterocolitica	Small and large intestine	Catarrhal enteritis.
Transmissible gastroenteritis virus (TGEV)	Small intestine	Obvious thin-walled small intestine (severe villous atrophy).
Porcine epidemic diarrhoea virus (PEDV)	Small intestine	Thin-walled small intestine (moderate villous atrophy).
Rotavirus, other viruses	Small intestine	Thin-walled small intestine (slight-to-moderate villous atrophy).
I. suis (occasionally other species in genus *Eimeria*)	Small intestine	Little evident gross lesions (catarrhal enteritis), but in severe cases, fibrinous-necrotising enteritis.
T. suis	Large intestine	Visible nematodes in the intestine lumen; muco-haemorrhagic enteritis.
Soybean meal hypersensitivity	Small intestine	Crypt hyperplasia and villous atrophy.

problem. The relatively late onset of the pro-blem and the sub-acute course suggested that this was not a post-weaning diarrhoea caused by the transition to a high-protein starter feed diet and probably not by very virulent agents such as TGEV either. The most common cau-ses of this type of problems are *L. intracellula-ris*, *E. coli*, *Brachyspira pilosicoli* among others.

Diagnostic approach and discussion

The most effective approach is to select a number of untreated 6-week old pigs (at least 2-3) showing deposition of soft faeces with undigested feed, euthanise them, and proceed to a detailed necropsy in order to record lesions that may provide information on the nature of the disease to be diagnosed. Considering the potential pathogens that may be involved, special attention should be given to the ileo-caecal valve area, colon and small intestine, as well as to the appearance of the mesenteric lymph nodes. Some samples of the small and large intestines (it is essential to include affected areas) should be selected and placed in adequately identified sterile jars. In parallel, other samples of intestine should be fixed in fresh buffered formalin (in a suffi-cient amount to cover the entire sample), with their ends tied off. The samples should be sent to the laboratory -fresh samples require refrigeration at 4 °C and should arrive at the laboratory in less than 24 h- indicating the anamnesis performed and the tests required.

For this case, a histopathological exami-nation and a bacteriological culture is the minimum that should be required from the laboratory. The use of a PCR test to confirm the presence of certain pathogens (*L. intrace-llularis*, *Brachyspira* spp.) or to determine viru-lence factors for isolated *E. coli* is advisable. If evidences of specific pathogens are obser-ved, further testing (table 2) can be required if available. In any case, it is a good idea to

request the laboratory to keep a frozen sam-ple (faeces or in some cases tissue) for further examination if needed.

The correct interpretation of the case requires the integration of the results obtai-ned using different techniques (microbiology, molecular biology, histopathology, etc.) and, particularly, the integrated interpretation of the lesions observed with the pathogens detec-ted. Often, more than one enteric pathogen is detected. While some of them (e. g. *E. coli* or *Salmonella* spp.) can be found in carrier pigs with no overt disease, others (e. g. TGEV) are not found in healthy weaners. For those that can be found in carriers, it is especially important to determine whether or not they were isolated abundantly in pure or almost pure culture, as well as if the lesions observed were compatible with these pathogens. On occasions, several enteric pathogens may co-circulate and one infection may follow another.

In the present case, considering the pre-vious differential diagnosis, the confirmation of proliferative ileitis (*L. intracellularis*), spiro-chetosis (*B. pilosicoli*) or colibacillosis (*E. coli*) should not be a problem if untreated animals are selected and, particularly, if PCR is used to confirm the results seen in the histopatho-logical analysis. The interpretation of negative results in treated animals is much more com-plicated and usually requires repeating the diagnosis with untreated individuals.

Analysis performed and results

Three six-week-old piglets were selected among those suffering from the condition and euthanised. Samples of small and large intes-tine (fresh segments with their ends tied off fixed in buffered formalin) were rapidly sent for diagnosis. Fixed samples were submitted for histopathological examination while fresh samples were used for direct observation, bac-teriology and molecular biology techniques. The initial visual examination of the intestines revealed an apparent thickening of the gut wall in the ileum. The mucosa was gently scraped and a small portion of faeces was suspended in sterile saline for its examination under a dark field microscope. No spirochaetes were observed.

Samples of intestinal content were seeded onto blood agar and MacConkey agar and incubated aerobically at 37 °C. In parallel, BJ agar plates (medium to grow *Brachyspira* spp.) were seeded and incubated under anaerobic conditions at 42 °C. A suspension of faeces retrieved from the ileum was used to determine the presence of *L. intracellularis*. An aliquot of faeces was kept at -80 °C. The histopathological examination revealed moderate hyperplasia of the ileal epithelium in the three selected animals. The bacteriological cultures yielded no relevant results (normal gut microbiota) while the PCR proved positive for *L. intracellularis* in all three cases and this pathogen was considered to be the cause of the process.

TABLE 2. Summary of laboratory tests for the diagnosis of the most common swine enteric diseases.

Cause	Preferred samples	1st election diagnostic approach	Observations	Complementary analyses
E. coli (ETEC and AEEC)	If possible, (proximal) small and large intestine of acutely affected animals; alternatively faeces.	Bacteriological culture + determination of type of fimbriae, enterotoxins, membrane virulence proteins intimin and EAST (usually by PCR).	Perform antibiogram. Negative results from appropriate samples [1] exclude colibacillosis.	Histopathology.
C. perfringens type C	Small intestine (jejunum) of euthanised or recently dead piglets.	Perform a smear of the intestine and Gram stain to observe the amount of clostridium-compatible bacteria + anaerobic culture + toxin determination (PCR).	Clostridia proliferate quickly after death. Simple isolation of *C. perfringens* is not enough.	Histopathology.
C. perfringens type A	Small intestine (jejunum) of euthanised or recently dead piglets.	Perform a smear of the intestine and Gram stain to observe the amount of clostridium-compatible bacteria + anaerobic culture + toxin determination (PCR).	Clostridia proliferate quickly after death. Simple isolation of *C. perfringens* is not enough.	Histopathology.

Continued ▶

TABLE 2. (Continuation). Summary of laboratory tests for the diagnosis of the most common swine enteric diseases.

Cause	Preferred samples	1st election diagnostic approach	Observations	Complementary analyses
C. difficile	Large bowel of euthanised or recently dead piglets.	Perform a smear of the intestine and Gram stain to observe the amount of clostridium-compatible bacteria + histopathology.	Signs, lesions and epidemiology are usually enough for diagnosis.	PCR (after bacteriological culture or directly from intestinal contents) to determine *C. difficile* toxins.
L. intracel-lularis	Ileum (ileocaecal valve).	Histopathology + determination of the presence of *L. intracellularis* (PCR, IHC, stains, etc.).	PCR from live animals is useful to detect infected animals but not to diagnose an outbreak.	Usually not performed although serological tests (ELISA) are available the market.
B. hyody-senteriae	Colon (and perhaps caecum) of euthanised or recently dead pigs. Faeces may be used if no losses occur.	PCR or a combination of anaerobic culture (42 °C) + PCR to increase sensitivity.	Treated animals may test negative in culture/PCR in spite of still being infected. Sensitivity using faeces is good in the event of a clinical outbreak with overt signs.	Histopathology, IHC, histological stains.
B. pilosicoli	Colon (and perhaps caecum) of euthanised pigs or alternatively faeces [2].	PCR or a combination of anaerobic culture (42 °C) + PCR to increase sensitivity.	Treated animals may test negative in culture/PCR in spite of still being infected. Sensitivity using faeces is good in the event of a clinical outbreak with overt signs.	Histopathology, IHC, histological stains.
Salmonella spp.	Large intestine, faeces.	Bacteriological culture + serotyping.	In cases of diarrhoea caused by *Salmonella*, the bacteria have to be isolated in primary (direct) cultures. Isolation after pre-enrichment + enrichment procedures is only an indication of a carrier status. Serology is useless to diagnose an outbreak.	Histopathology, PCR.

Continued ▶

TABLE 2. (Continuation). Summary of laboratory tests for the diagnosis of the most common swine enteric diseases.

Cause	Preferred samples	1st election diagnostic approach	Observations	Complementary analyses
Y. entero-colitica	Small and large intestine.	Bacteriological culture + serotyping.	There are carriers.	Usually not performed.
TGEV	Small intestine of acutely affected animals or recently dead pigs; alternatively faeces.	Histopathology + Capture ELISA or PCR.	The virus may disappear rapidly from faeces in recovering animals.	Usually not performed although serological tests (ELISA) exist in the market.
PEDV	Small intestine of acutely affected animals or recently dead pigs; alternatively faeces.	Histopathology + Capture ELISA or PCR.	The virus may disappear rapidly from faeces in recovering animals.	Usually not performed.
Rotavirus, other viruses	Small intestine of acutely affected animals or recently dead pigs; alternatively faeces.	Histopathology + Capture ELISA or PCR.	The virus may disappear rapidly from faeces in recovering animals.	Usually not performed.
I. suis	Faeces, alternatively small intestine of piglets in the affected batch [3] (3-5 pigs/litter, sampling 5-10 litters at the 2nd-3rd week of age).	Flotation, smears of the small intestine [4] + histopathology.	Oocysts are not detected in faeces during the acute phase of coccidiosis in neonates; subsequently even formed faeces can be positive.	Usually not performed.
T. suis	Large intestine or faeces.	Flotation, observation of parasites in the bowel after a necropsy.	Often, shedding of T. suis in faeces is not constant or even sporadic.	Usually not performed.
Soy bean meal hyper-sensitivity	Small intestine.	Histopathology.	Most often diagnosed by changing the diet after ruling out other potential causes.	Usually not performed.

[1] In the context of this table, appropriate samples refer to those obtained from correctly selected animals, shipped in appropriate conditions to the laboratory. See other chapters of this book for more details.

[2] B. pilosicoli rarely causes the death of the pig or a very severe disease.

[3] Sensitivity is not increased by sampling diarrhoeic pigs alone.

[4] In the primary acute phase it could be necessary to euthanise some of the affected piglets.

7

Laboratory diagnosis of systemic disorders

INTRODUCTION

Disorders and diseases involving several organic systems are sometimes difficult to differentiate from those affecting a specific one (respiratory and digestive problems, mainly). Even if a disorder is multisystemic, its manifestation is usually dominated by one main clinical sign rather than by multiple signs. This is generally true on an individual basis, but certainly varies within a population of diseased pigs. Apart from the obvious finding of widespread organic damage such as fibrinous polyserositis or generalised haemorrhages, the observation of different signs and/or gross lesions in a group of pigs at the same time is highly suggestive of a systemic disease affecting the immune system. Acquired immunological disorders are good examples of how the clinical and pathological signs of a particular problem can vary, and of the lack of a proper response to antibiotics. Moreover, in the latter case, the likelihood of concomitant infections favoured by immune dysfunction makes the establishment of a clear-cut diagnosis of the primary condition more difficult, and the veterinary surgeon's work is usually based on the most obvious clinical signs.

Most systemic diseases in pigs are of infectious/contagious aetiology and, therefore, the vet's first reaction is usually to search for potential causative agents. However, it should be highlighted that toxic and nutritional disorders can also cause systemic problems. Although they are generally perceived as population disorders, systemic problems may be an individual problem (e. g. multiple abscesses due to neonatal umbilical infections or infections secondary to tail biting). In these cases, the number of affected pigs within a batch should be much more limited (one or a few animals).

Finally, it is important to note that a number of disorders included in this chapter are also addressed in other sections of this guide. Therefore, this chapter will concentrate on those conditions with evident multiple organ affection, both from a clinical and a pathological point of view.

CLINICAL EXAMINATION

It is difficult to define specific clinical signs that are indicative of an unequivocal systemic disorder. A multiple organ dysfunction is usually suspected when pigs become ill or "do poorly" without a specific predominant clinical sign in the studied batch. These animals may be lethargic, depressed, anorexic, febrile, dehydrated and/or prostrate, with variable morbidity and mortality rates.

On clinical examination, there are external findings that may strongly suggest certain systemic disorders, although a proper differential diagnosis list must be established. A summary of these conditions is displayed in table 1. For example, generalised cutaneous haemorrhages are the consequence of a systemic damage, but their origin can greatly vary depending on the causative condition (infectious disease, toxicity, immunological disorder, etc.). Further investigations are thus needed to establish the aetiology of multiple skin haemorrhages.

PATHOLOGICAL ASSESSMENT

The clinical presentation of systemic disorders can be either hyperacute, acute or subacute. It will be easier for the veterinary surgeon to diagnose the potential cause with the two latter cases, since a number of potential gross lesions can be documented during the necropsy (table 2). Although, samples for microbiological, virological, serological, molecular biology and toxicological analyses may be collected depending on the established clinical-pathological suspicions, additional laboratory tests will usually give better results in acute-subacute clinical pictures than in chronic stages.

TABLE 1. External findings leading to suspicion of a systemic disorder.

External sign	Concomitant signs	Suspected condition/s
Cutaneous diamond-shaped lesions	Fever, prostration	Erysipelas
Cutaneous irregular-shaped lesions	Prostration, no fever, lethargy, sometimes no other signs	Porcine dermatitis and nephropathy syndrome
Poor body condition, rough hair	Variable, depending on the specific cause	PCV2-SD, PRRS, PFTS, others
Generalised cyanosis	Fever, prostration, dehydration	Bacterial septicaemia
Multiple swollen joints	Fever, lameness, prostration-sometimes, central nervous signs	Bacterial septicaemia

TABLE 2. Pathological findings at necropsy suggestive of systemic disorders, potential generic aetiology and evolution stage in pigs.

Pathological finding	Suspected generic aetiology	Evolution stage
Generalised haemorrhages	Bacteria, virus, immunological	Acute
Generalised oedema	Bacteria (toxins), severe liver damage of other origin	Acute, chronic
Fibrinous/purulent polyarthritis	Bacteria	Acute, subacute
Proliferative/fibrous polyarthritis	Bacteria	Chronic
Fibrinous polyserositis	Bacteria	Acute, subacute
Fibrous polyserositis	Bacteria	Chronic
Necrotic foci in parenchymatous organs	Virus	Acute
Serous atrophy of fat	Catabolic condition of different origin	Chronic
Thrombotic valvular endocarditis	Bacteria	Chronic
Splenomegaly	Bacteria, virus, immunological	Acute
Generalised lymphadenopathy	Bacteria, virus	Acute, subacute
Generalised abscesses	Bacteria	Subacute, chronic

DIFFERENTIAL DIAGNOSES

They are organised in different sections depending on the age and production stage of the animals. The differential diagnoses of suckling piglets, growing and finishing pigs and adults will therefore be explained according to the clinical signs, lesions, aetiologies and laboratory techniques.

Suckling piglets

An algorithm diagnostic of the main systemic disorders in suckling pigs based on clinical signs, lesions and laboratory techniques is shown in figure 1.

Dyspnoea is rarely observed in newborn piglets and is usually attributed to a congenital PRRSV infection when affecting a significant number of animals. The affected piglets usually display enlarged lymph nodes (generalised lymphadenopathy). More information about PRRSV is included in chapter 5. Several possibilities should be included in the differential diagnosis. When dyspnoea affects random animals or simply one, other causes such as diaphragmatic hernia or rib fracture due to crushing by the sow should be considered. However, respiratory problems in suckling pigs are more frequent in the second and third weeks of age. Their aetiology is usually bacterial and *Pasteurella multocida* and *Bordetella bronchiseptica* are the most frequent causative agents. Nonetheless, these specifically respiratory bacterial problems do not mean that PRRSV may not also be involved.

Sudden death is quite a non-specific sign, but may be the perceived typical sign of a very fast evolving condition such as septicaemia, or of a viral infection such as that caused by the pseudorabies virus. Sporadically, this latter disease can present as necrotic foci on the surface of organs such as the liver, kidneys or spleen.

Joint swelling as a result of bacterial septicaemia (together or not with fibrinous polyserositis/meningitis) is discussed in the section covering the differential diagnosis in "growing and finishing pigs". **Fever** is usually present during bacteraemia, viraemia and in the acute phase of serosal inflammation. Obviously, fever is quite a non-specific sign and other non-systemic conditions can also cause it.

Hypoglycaemia may result from several factors affecting the sow such as poor nutrition, the presence of a disease, agalaxia, a cold or chilly environment and/or any disease in the piglet that impairs suckling. More information on this condition as well as on **hypoxia** is provided in chapter 9.

Some seldom occurring findings that lead to suspicion of systemic infections are greyish-white foci in the kidneys, usually associated with reproductive disorders caused by *Leptospira* spp., or petechial haemorrhages in kidneys due to erysipelas. In both cases, the isolation of the bacterial agent would confirm the presumptive diagnosis. Neonatal isoerythrolysis is another condition that is sometimes observed. It is manifested by jaundice and multiple cutaneous and systemic haemorrhages due to colostrum containing antibodies against pig erythrocytes.

Growing and finishing pigs

A diagnostic algorithm of the main systemic disorders in growing and finishing pigs based on clinical signs, lesions and laboratory techniques is presented in figure 2.

Poor body condition is a very generic symptom of some systemic and non-systemic diseases, as well as of management problems. Therefore, this sign must be accompanied by thorough clinical and epidemiological investigations on the farm, assessing the presence of fever and other concomitant signs. Recently, a disease named periweaning failure-to-thrive syndrome (PFTS) has been described as a progressive loss of body condition in recently weaned piglets. At necropsy, almost no significant gross lesions are observed besides those typical of a catabolic process (serous atrophy of fat, thymus atrophy, etc.). As of today, its aetiology is not precisely known, and ruling out known infectious diseases as well as nutritional, environmental and management causes is the way to establish a presumptive diagnosis.

FIGURE 1. Main differential diagnoses in suckling pigs suffering from systemic disorders.

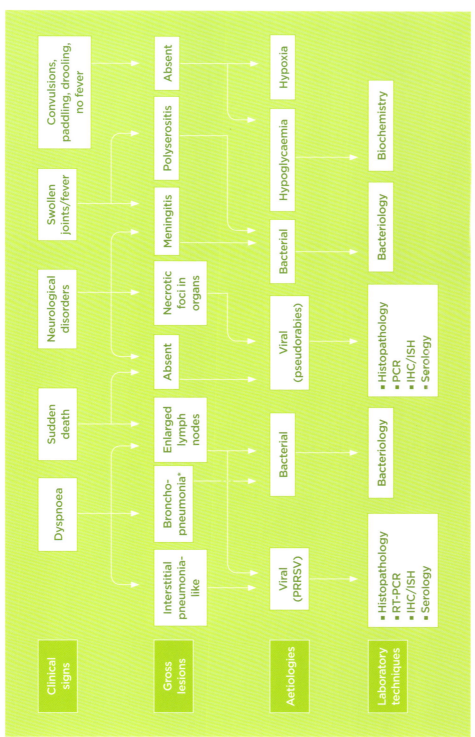

*Bacterial bronchopneumonia is not a systemic problem, but it is frequently found in PRRSV infected pigs.

FIGURE 2. Main differential diagnoses in growing-finishing pigs suffering from systemic disorders.

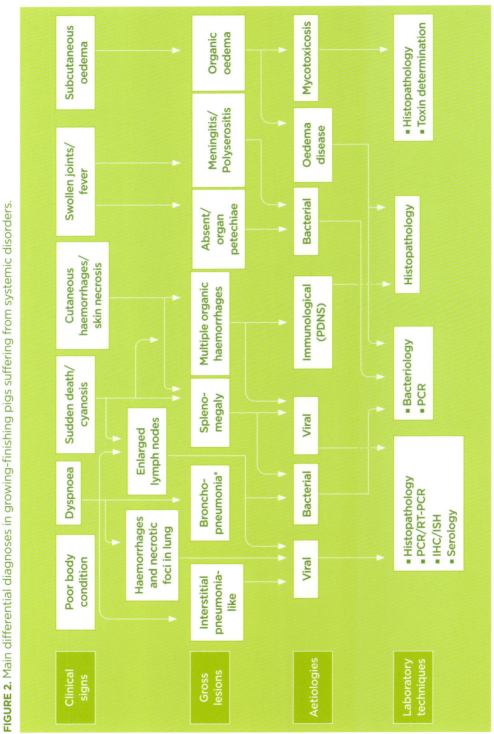

*Bacterial bronchopneumonia is not a systemic problem, but it is frequently found in pigs infected by viruses.

Dyspnoea is a frequent finding in growing/finishing pigs and PRRSV is one of its most common causes (see chapter 5). The animals suffering from dyspnoea usually display lymphadenopathy. Respiratory problems together with generalised lymphadenopathy are the typical features of porcine circovirus type 2-systemic disease (PCV2-SD). This condition is rarely seen nowadays because of widespread vaccination against PCV2, but a definitive diagnosis should be established by means of a histopathological examination of the lymphoid tissues (moderate to severe lymphocyte depletion and granulomatous inflammation) and virus detection in these lesions (moderate to high amount of PCV2 antigen or genome). Several possibilities should be included in the differential diagnosis. In both scenarios, PRRS and PCV2-SD, the presence of concomitant respiratory infections that worsen the clinical picture is usual. The bacteria most frequently associated with these are *Mycoplasma hyopneumoniae, P. multocida, B. bronchiseptica* and *Streptococcus* spp. Although they are seldom observed, necrotic foci in the lungs and lung haemorrhages are very suggestive of pseudorabies infection.

Sudden death is, again, quite a non-specific sign, but it can be observed as a consequence of a bacterial systemic infection, with or without lymphadenopathy and/or splenomegaly. **Cyanosis and multiple petechiae** in organs, mainly in the kidneys, and the absence of other gross lesions are very suggestive of bacterial septicaemia (it is important to take erysipelas into account) or of a viral infection caused by hyperacute presentations of classical or african swine fever. However, in addition to the possibility of sudden death, the most obvious clinical signs of erysipelas and swine fevers are cutaneous and organic haemorrhages. Special attention should be paid to lymph node haemorrhages in african swine fever. Moreover, porcine dermatitis and nephropathy syndrome

(PDNS), an immune complex disease (see chapter 10), can easily be confused with swine fevers from a pathological point of view. A relatively easy way of differentiating PDNS from African and classical swine fevers is by determining the urea and creatinin levels in serum; the values of PDNS-affected pigs are, usually, above the normal levels (> 65 mg/dl for urea and > 2.5 mg/dl for creatinin), these values sometimes being very high. Therefore, it is crucial to establish a clear-cut list of conditions involving cutaneous and systemic haemorrhages; finally, communication with the health authorities is recommended.

Swollen joints and **fever** are typical of systemic bacterial diseases, mainly in their acute phase. In a number of cases, this clinical picture can be pathologically described as fibrinous-purulent polyarthritis, with or without accompanying fibrinous polyserositis. The most common causative agents are *Haemophilus parasuis* and *Streptococcus suis*, but *Mycoplasma hyorhinis* should be seriously considered in the differential diagnosis list. Although it is less common, *Escherichia coli* may also be involved. Meningitis may be a manifestation of septicaemia caused by both *H. parasuis* and *S. suis*. A chronification of these lesions generally causes fibrous polyserositis, arthritis and periarthritis. A diagnostic approach in chronic stages is usually useless.

Subcutaneous oedema is rather typical of oedema disease (caused by enterotoxigenic *E. coli*). There is usually oedema of in the eyelids and face (naso-facial oedema) and of the gastric wall and mesocolon. The definitive diagnosis can be established by histopathological analysis of the brain, since a symmetric bilateral polioencephalomalacia of the brainstem is considered pathognomonic for this disease. An intestinal bacteriological analysis would be also recommended, since it is important to note that the bacteria are strictly located in the intestine and that their pathological effect is caused by their toxins. The differential diagnosis of generalised oedema would be chronic liver damage leading to decreased oncotic pressure due to mycotoxicosis (aflatoxicosis), mulberry heart disease or cardiac insufficiency causing chronic passive congestion.

Sows and boars
Systemic diseases are not frequent in adult pigs, although the same diseases as those indicated for finishing pigs may apply. Specifically, erysipelas and other bacterial septicaemias are the most frequent systemic problems affecting sows and boars. However, bacteria such as *S. suis* or *H. parasuis* rarely cause diseases in adults, unless the infected pigs' immune system is naïve to these agents. Other conditions cited in the previous section are of lesser severity in adults or simply do not occur in standard conditions (again, due to their immunological status or because of age-dependent resistance). The effect of PRRSV in adults, and specifically pregnant sows, is included in chapter 8. The infection of naïve adult pigs with African and classical swine fever may resemble that observed for growing/finishing pigs.

CLINICAL CASE

Clinical history
Farrow-to-finish, 200-sow farm with a continuous flow production system. A significant number of animals with growth retardation were observed. The clinical history included a severe episode of tail and ear biting in growing/finishing pigs in the previous year. Subsequently, a mortality problem due to central nervous clinical signs appeared in early nursery pigs. No definitive diagnosis was established, but the suspicion included streptococcal meningitis and oedema disease; the use of colistin in the feed improved the clinical picture, so the latter condition was considered to be the cause

of the problem. Thereafter, a clinical picture of growth retardation (fig. 3), dyspnoea and increased mortality affected late nursery and early fattening pigs; sporadic diarrhoea was also observed. The mortality of the affected batch finally reached 20%. The pigs on the farm were regularly vaccinated against pseudorabies virus. A PCV2 vaccine was not available at the time when this case occurred.

Pathological analysis
At necropsy, three live and one dead 3-month-old, male pigs (of 10 kg approx.) showed evident growth retardation (marked dorsal spine and rough hair) and respiratory distress. The four pigs showed a lack of pulmonary collapse, randomly distributed multifocal areas of parenchymal consolidation (fig. 4) and generalised lymphadenopathy. Two of them showed cranioventral pulmonary consolidation (catarrhal-purulent bronchopneumonia). One displayed fibrinous pericarditis and pleuritis and another pig presented with fibrous pleuritis. One of them also showed gastric ulceration of the pars esophagea. Histopathologically, the four pigs showed moderate to severe lymphocyte depletion with granulomatous inflammation of the lymphoid tissues, mainly in the lymph nodes (fig. 5), tonsil and Peyer's patches. Moreover, all the pigs suffered from subacute interstitial pneumonia. Mild lympho-histiocytic hepatitis was also observed in 3 animals and slight subacute interstitial nephritis in one of them.

Laboratory analyses
The pathological diagnoses pointed to PCV2-SD and this was confirmed by the finding of moderate to high amounts of PCV2 nucleic acid in the lymphatic tissues (fig. 6). A RT-PCR test to detect PRRSV was also carried out on serum samples and one of the pigs was positive. No further laboratory analyses were performed.

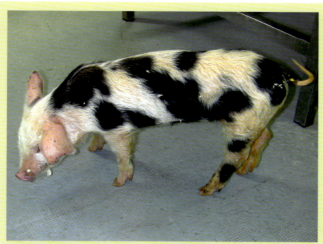

Figure 3. Pig showing poor body condition in a relatively chronic stage. In general terms, the animal selected to be analysed for PCV2-SD should ideally be one with no more than 1 week of clinical evolution.

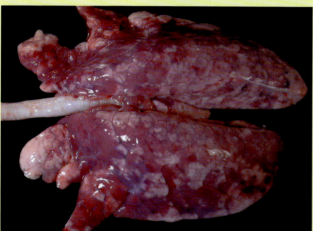

Figure 4. Lung. Lack of pulmonary collapse together with a lobular pattern; very slight evidence of interstitial oedema. These three gross characteristics are highly suggestive of subacute interstitial pneumonia, typical of viral infections.

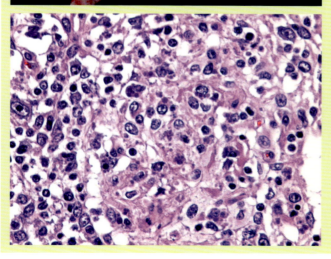

Figure 5. Lymph node, HE stain. Moderate lymphocyte depletion and granulomatous inflammation of the lymph node parenchyma. The central area corresponds to a lymphoid follicle, which contains macrophages showing round intracytoplasmic inclusion bodies typical of PCV2.

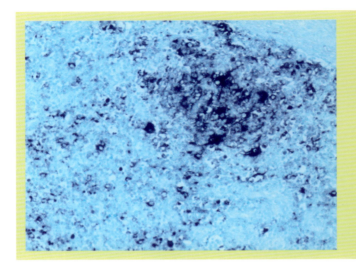

Figure 6. Lymph node, PCV2 *in situ* hybridisation. Moderate amount of PCV2 nucleic acid (stained in blue) contained in the cytoplasm of macrophages and multinucleated giant cells.

Discussion

This is a typical case of laboratory-confirmed PCV2-SD with a concomitant infection by PRRSV. Although the clinical picture was already suggestive of these conditions (one, the other or both viruses), it was important to establish a definitive diagnosis. At the time of this case, no PCV2 vaccine was available and it was important to get a diagnosis of the condition. If PCV2-SD had been ruled out, potential counteracting actions would have been established, mainly taking into account PRRSV and concomitant bacterial respiratory infections. It is important to note, however, that the lack of a definitive PCV2-SD laboratory diagnosis does not necessarily rule out the condition. Making an appropriate selection of animals is paramount; it must include pigs that are representative of the disease problem, which implies choosing pigs in the early stages of the condition and avoiding the necropsy and sampling of chronically affected pigs. In the current context, animals would receive PCV2 vaccine around weaning age. However, at that time, the solution that offered the best result was a change in the genetic background of the boars, but the condition lasted for more than one year with nursery-growing mortality rates varying between 10 and 30% in each batch. Management practices were also improved, but the farm had been built in the 60s and was thus very old so the possibility of changing the animal flow was not considered due to economic constraints.

8

Laboratory diagnosis of reproductive disorders

INTRODUCTION

The diagnosis of reproductive disorders is a difficult process that requires an extended and systematic clinical and laboratory approach. In some cases, a final diagnosis is not achieved, and this process may seem exhausting or disappointing. In this scenario, it is important to keep in mind that reproduction can be influenced by a number of infectious and non-infectious factors. Among the latter ones, the housing, the environment, genetics, nutrition and management are important factors to consider; moreover, one problem may often give rise to others. For example, the diagnostic success rate for sporadic abortions is about 50%, being greater in outbreaks. For these reasons, the diagnosis of reproductive failure requires an open mind and special attention to data records, clinical observation, pathological examination and laboratory testing. Hence, the diagnosis of reproductive failure requires the collection of reliable information and its use in a meaningful way.

Reproductive failure in sows can occur during anoestrus, ovulation and ova production, fertilisation and implantation, as well as during the last two thirds of gestation (foetal death) or at farrowing (stillborn piglets). In general, but especially for the first four physiological phases, it is important to have a basic knowledge of the normal reproductive physiology of sows and boars to deal with a reproductive disorder. There is a lot of information available in the literature on porcine reproductive physiology and endocrinology and the management, clinical assessment and treatment of reproductive failure; this chapter will therefore mainly focus on reproductive diagnosis from a laboratory point of view.

DATA ANALYSIS AND CLINICAL EXAMINATION

In many cases, the cause of reproductive failure is a non-infectious process. Therefore, the **analysis of data records** and the assessment of the biological performance of the breeding herd is a first step when dealing with a reproductive problem. The information related to fertility, lactation performance, the interval from entry or weaning to mating and to piglet survival until weaning should be carefully examined. Subsequently, an inspection of the environment of the farm, its facilities management, the health status of the pigs, epidemiological data, and nutrition may suggest one or several factors as a cause of the reproductive failure. **The clinical examination** of the animals, together with the pathological assessment, is a useful tool to rule out a systemic problem and make sure the failure is associated with a reproductive cause. For example, it is essential to find out if the aborting sows have or have had clinical signs or a systemic illness, either or near the time of abortion. If this is the case, samples from the sow and foetuses may be submitted for laboratory analyses. However, the nature of the sow's illness should be also established in order to choose an appropriate sampling strategy. It is necessary to keep in mind that some infectious (e. g. swine influenza, erysipelas) and non-infectious diseases (e. g. seasonal infertility) do not affect the foetuses, but may cause fever or stress in the sow that could predispose to abortion. In these cases, the laboratory analyses of the foetuses will be unsuccessful.

PATHOLOGICAL ASSESSMENT

The analysis of the different factors that affect **boars** is also important for successful reproductive diagnosis. Some of these factors are related to the age of the animal, the presence of systemic or reproductive diseases, the frequency of mating and quality of the semen, among others. Semen evaluation to determine the initial quality of a boar ejaculate is usually performed on the farm or at the boar stud. The description of the parameters for semen evaluation is beyond the objectives of this chapter. However, there are some specific pathogens that can infect the testicular parenchyma and disrupt spermatogenesis. These are *Brucella* spp., *Chlamydophila* spp., Japanese B encephalitis virus and porcine rubulavirus (blue eye disease virus). Other infectious agents can elicit a fever response without infecting the testicles and subsequently affect spermatogenesis (e. g. erysipelas or swine influenza). Moreover, epididymal, testicular or scrotal damage of a non-infectious cause can also cause testicular degeneration and atrophy of the organ.

From a diagnostic point of view, once fertilisation has occurred, **pregnancy failure** is divided into three stages depending on the foetal development and potential viability: early embryonic mortality (approximately before 30-35 days after fecundation), foetal loss (abortion) and stillbirth. Some of the most common infectious and toxic causes of embryonic death, abortion and stillbirth are shown in table 1. Moreover, there are many non-infectious factors than can lead to reproductive failure in these phases. Some of them are related to the management of the sows, genetics, nutrition, the boar effect, the farrow-to-service interval, the litter size, ambient temperature and season, among others.

Embryonic death produces return to oestrus at a normal or delayed interval depending on the moment of death. In these cases, the embryos are reabsorbed or expulsed with minimal or no changes in the reproductive tract of the sow. Identifying the cause of embryonic loss is difficult because there rarely are embryonic or placental tissues to examine.

Abortion means the expulsion of the foetus before the end of gestation. The foetus may be fresh, autolytic, mummified or macerated. The grade of autolysis depends on the time elapsed after foetal death. **Mummification** implies an advanced degree of autolysis and is the consequence of foetal retention during long periods of time; the foetuses are dehydrated and become firm, dry masses covered by leathery skin. There is an absence of lytic bacteria and it is usually attributed to viral infections, such as PPV. **Maceration** occurs when the foetus decomposes due to the presence of bacteria in the uterus; these bacteria could be the cause of foetal death or a subsequent contamination entered via the cervix.

Stillbirth occurs when the foetus dies a few days before or during parturition (no lung inflation-no flotation in liquid). This terminology is sometimes also used when the piglet dies shortly (a few hours) after birth. However, if there is partial lung inflation (it would float in liquid), it should be considered as post-birth death (perinatal mortality).

TABLE 1. Most common infectious and toxic causes of infertility, embryonic death, abortion and stillbirths in pigs.

	Infertility	Embryonic death	Abortion	Stillbirth
Infectious				
PRRSV			X	X
PCV2		X	X	X
PPV		X		X
ADV		X	X	X
SIV	X		X	X
EMCV			X	X
Enterovirus/Teschovirus	X	X	X	X
CSFV		X	X	X
Leptospira spp.	X		X	
Brucella spp.	X		X	
Toxoplasma gondii			X	X
Toxic				
Carbon monoxide			X	X
Zearalenone	X	X		

DIFFERENTIAL DIAGNOSES

From an epidemiological point of view, it is useful to establish the approximate age at which the foetus died. This can be calculated by measuring the length from the crown of the head to the tail base (in centimetres) and applying the following formula:

$$\text{Days of gestation} = (\text{length} \times 3) + 21$$

In case of abortion or stillbirth, the analysis of the foetus and placenta can be useful to confirm or rule out an infectious aetiology. Figure 1 summarises the lesions that can be observed in foetuses and membranes and their possible causes. Nevertheless, gross foetal or placental lesions in pigs are rarely observed; therefore, a systematic collection of samples for laboratory examination is necessary.

Malformations are usually attributed to viral infections such as classical swine fever, plant or drug toxicity and some genetic traits. These foetal anomalies consist of arthrogryposis, palatoschisis (cleft palate) and nervous system malformations (e. g. cerebellar hypoplasia).

The scant presence of fibrinous **exudates, necrosis or haemorrhages** on the surface of the viscera or placenta is suggestive of bacterial infection (*Streptococcus* spp., *E. coli*, *A. pyogenes*, *Staphylococcus* spp., etc.). Microscopically, the observation of purulent lesions in the lungs or other organs is suggestive of bacterial infection. **Icterus** is characteristic of leptospirosis, but is an uncommon finding.

FIGURE 1. Foetal and placental lesions related to possible aetiologies and their diagnostic procedures.

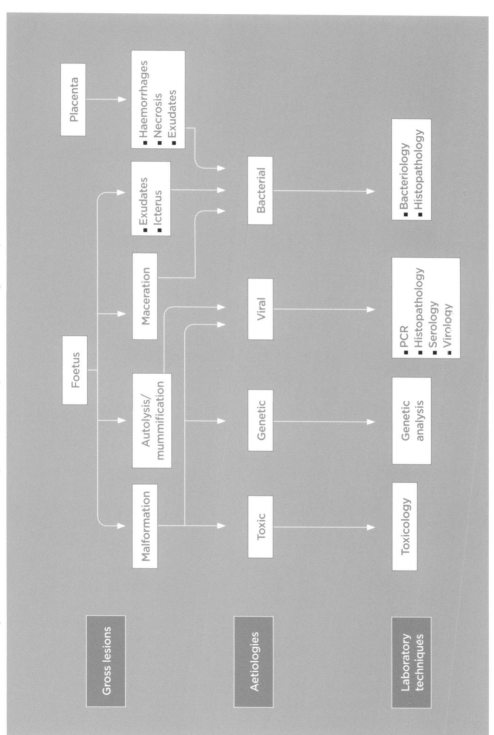

Viral infections (PRRSV, PCV2, PPV, ADV, SIV, etc.) usually appear as outbreaks and cause similar reproductive manifestations such as late-term abortions, stillbirths and weak-born pigs, with an absence of gross lesions in most cases. In these scenarios, the presence of microscopic lesions such as those of non-suppurative encephalitis, myocarditis, interstitial pneumonia or multifocal necrotising lesions are rather suggestive of viral infection.

One of the most common **toxicoses** is carbon monoxide toxicity, related with an inadequate combustion of fuels in heated facilities; foetuses show a cherry-red colouration of the organs and confirmation is made by detection of carboxyhaemoglobin levels > 2% in foetal thoracic fluid. Zearalenone is an estrogenic mycotoxin present in the feed and is associated with persistent oestrus (vulvar tumefaction), infertility and embryonic death.

COLLECTION OF SAMPLES

When investigating a case of pregnancy failure, the clinician may decide to take samples for laboratory testing after studying the records and carrying out a clinical and pathological examination. These samples will depend on the hypothesis on the cause of the problem. It is recommended to contact the laboratory in advance since each one has specific protocols. General guidelines on how to collect and submit samples to the laboratory were given in chapter 2. This section provides more detailed information regarding sample taking in case of reproductive problems.

When an infectious disease is suspected, maternal, placental and foetal factors must be considered. In case of abortion, the examination and proper sampling of the **foetus and placenta** are essential to obtain a successful diagnosis. When possible, the submission of weak, live neonates is useful to get as many fresh samples as possible. If not, several whole foetuses with placentas should be submitted for laboratory examination (fig. 2). Mummified foetuses are usually not suitable for testing, except for porcine parvovirus (PPV) and *T. gondii*. Moreover, maternal samples must also be collected to rule out any infectious agent that may not be found in the foetuses.

Serology is sometimes useful to detect specific infections in the sow. However, the results depend on the time elapsed between the infection and the occurrence of abortion. Fourteen or more days post-infection are usually needed to detect seroconversion (see chapter 4). Therefore, in the case of an abortion due to an acute infectious systemic illness, paired serum samples may demonstrate a rise in the antibody titre related to the abortion. The foetuses infected after 70 days of gestation are able to develop an antibody response; hence, a positive result confirms the diagnosis. In foetuses, thoracic fluid can be used for antibody detection purposes.

CLINICAL CASE

Clinical history
In an intensive farrowing farm of 400 sows, 40 sows had had sporadic abortions at different stages of gestation in the last 6 weeks. Apart from this group, 20 sows had had vaginal discharge around 20 days post-breeding. After abortion, the sows did not get pregnant, at least on the first heat cycle. The vet prescribed an antibiotic treatment, but it was unsuccessful; a viral infection was thus suspected, and several aborted foetuses were submitted to laboratory diagnosis.

Laboratory examination
Four foetuses from the same litter, aborted at the third month of gestation, were submitted for laboratory investigations (fig. 3). In

FIGURE 2. Guidelines for sample collection in case of reproductive failure.

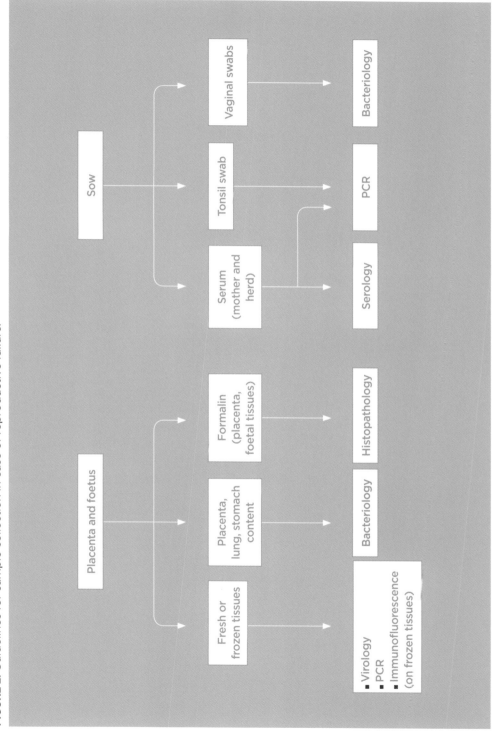

two foetuses, the gross inspection of the chorion (foetal placenta) revealed the presence of multifocal areas of necrosis with scant fibrinous-purulent exudate. Histopathologically, these corresponded to multiple foci of necrosis of the trophoblast with severe neutrophilic infiltration (fig. 4). One of the animals also showed neutrophilic infiltration in the pulmonary alveoli; a Gram stain revealed the presence of intralesional Gram-negative bacteria. No gross or histopathological lesions were observed in the other two foetuses. *In situ* hybridisation (ISH) for PCV2 and immunohistochemistry (IHC) for PRRSV yielded negative results in all the cases. A bacteriological examination was performed from the gastric content of all the foetuses and *Brucella suis* was isolated from one of the piglets with placental lesions.

Discussion

In this case, the pathological results suggested a bacterial infection as the cause of the abortions. Bacteriology confirmed the presence of *B. suis* in one of the foetuses and it was therefore considered to be the causative agent of that particular abortion. It is very likely that this pathogen was the aetiology of the general reproductive failure observed on the farm. The fact that these bacteria were only isolated from one foetus confirms the importance of submitting several foetuses for laboratory diagnosis. Although molecular or virology techniques were not performed, the absence of compatible microscopic lesions, together with the negative results obtained with ISH and IHC, suggested that a viral agent was not apparently involved in these cases.

When *B. suis* first enters a herd of naïve animals, it rapidly spreads among the animals. The clinical signs are usually abortions, increased perinatal mortality and infertility. However, most of the infected non-gestating sows do not exhibit clinical signs. On the other hand, the infection in boars can cause different degrees of severity of orchitis and epididymitis, sometimes with a marked increase of testicle size and necrotising inflammation with mineralisation of the testis parenchyma (fig. 5). In this particular case, the source of infection was not identified, but it may be speculated that the introduction of infected live animals, the contact with infected wildlife reservoirs and artificial insemination with semen from infected boars are the most probable origins.

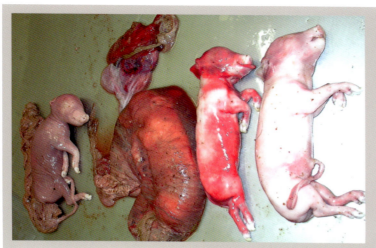

Figure 3. Aborted foetuses from the same litter. The first and third from the left show autolytic changes (oedema, congestion).

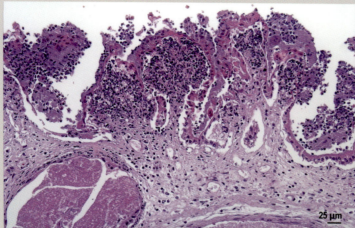

Figure 4. Chorion from an aborted foetus. There is multifocal to diffuse, severe necrosis of the trophoblast with neutrophilic infiltration.

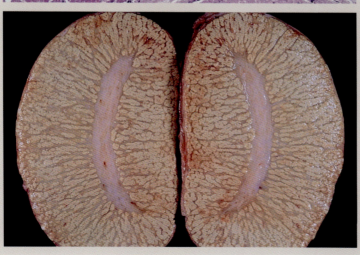

Figure 5. Testicle cut in two halves. Marked increase in size of a testicle, which shows a generalised necrosis of the parenchyma (necrotising orchitis).

9

Laboratory diagnosis of nervous and locomotor disorders

INTRODUCTION

Disorders and diseases involving the nervous and locomotor systems are rather common in the swine industry. However, they are usually observed as individual problems with occasional herd outbreaks. Most nervous disorders are of sudden onset or acute outbreaks that may be infectious or of toxic origin. In contrast, many bone alterations are chronic disorders involving a defective formation of the skeletal structures or the effects of a chronic infection or trauma. In addition, most musculoskeletal disorders are difficult to differentiate only by clinical examination.

It is should be highlighted that the diseases affecting either the nervous or locomotor systems often have similar general clinical presentations. Hence, in order to perform an accurate diagnostic investigation, the veterinary clinician must collect a detailed clinical history including past and present history, clinical inspection, environmental assessment and individual pathological examination. The floors, equipment, interaction with humans and other pigs all contribute to locomotor disorders. It is also important to differentiate the clinical problems on the basis of the age of the affected population. Thus, these disorders can be classified according to whether they affect newborn and suckling piglets, growing and finishing pigs, and adults.

CLINICAL EXAMINATION

Identifying the clinical signs is fundamental to locate the problem anatomically, select samples and diagnose the clinical disease. A precise definition of the problem is particularly important in nervous and musculosketal problems; therefore, some neurological terms that are frequently used to refer to nervous and locomotor disorders are given in table 1.

TABLE 1. Neurological terms and sample selection in cases of nervous and/or locomotor system disorders.

Term	Definition	Anatomic location of injury				
		Brain	SC	Nerves	Muscles	Other
Ataxia	Failure of movement coordination.	X	X		X	
Circling	Moving in circles.	X		CN VIII		Internal ear
Coma	A state of unconsciousness in which the animal does not respond to painful stimuli.	X				
Convulsion/seizures	Episode of violent involuntary contraction of muscles and altered consciousness.	X				Blood
Facial deficits	Facial sensory and motion alterations.			CN V, VII		
Fasciculation	Small local involuntary muscular contraction visible under the skin.		X	PN	X	Blood

Continued ▶

TABLE 1. (Continuation). Neurological terms and sample selection in cases of nervous and/or locomotor system disorders.

Term	Definition	Anatomic location of injury				
		Brain	SC	Nerves	Muscles	Other
Flaccidity	Lack of muscular tone.		X	PN		
Head-pressing	Forward walking interrupted when the animal touches a fixed object and pushes its head against it.	X				
Head-tilt	Turn of the head along the animal's central axis to one side or the other.	X		CN VIII		
Hemiparesis	Decreased motor function of the limbs of one side of the body.	X	X			
Hemiplegia	Paralysis of the limbs of one side of the body.	X	X			
Hyperesthesia	Excessive sensitivity to a normal level of stimulation in a particular area.		X		X	
Monoparesis	Decreased motor function of a single limb.		X	PN		
Nystagmus	Rhythmic oscillating movements of the eye.	X		CN VIII		
Paddling	A movement similar to kicking or paddling with the legs.	X				
Paraplegia	Paralysis of the rear half of the body.		X			
Paraparesis	Decreased motor function of the rear half of the body.		X			
Propioceptive deficits	Improper position of limbs and feet. Abnormal postural reactions.	X	X	PN		
Spasticity/ rigidity	Increased muscular tone or stiffness.	X	X	PN	X	
Tetraplegia	Paralysis of all four limbs		X	PN		
Tremor	Involuntary trembling, shaking.	X	X	PN		
Vestibular syndrome	A group of symptoms consisting of circling, loss of balance, head-tilt, nystagmus, recumbency and/or paddling.	X		CN VIII		Internal ear
Vision deficits			X		CN II	Eye

CN: cranial nerves; PN: peripheral nerves; SC: spinal cord.

PATHOLOGICAL ASSESSMENT

In the absence of significant lesions, it is necessary to perform a systematic collection of samples from the brain, spinal cord, peripheral nerves, bones, muscles and joints for histopathological examination. Moreover, samples for microbiological, virological, serological, molecular biology and toxicological analyses might also be collected depending on the clinical suspicions established. Table 2 summarises the most frequent pathological problems that are usually used to define the different alterations of the nervous and musculoskeletal systems.

DIFFERENTIAL DIAGNOSES

They are organised in different sections depending on the age and production stage of the animals. The differential diagnoses in suckling piglets, growing and finishing pigs and adults will be explained according to the clinical symptoms, lesions, aetiologies and laboratory techniques. Malformations of the nervous and locomotor system observed in foetuses are explained in chapter 8.

TABLE 2. Pathological terms used to describe lesions in the nervous and locomotor system.

Term	Definition
Arthritis	Inflammation of a joint.
Diskospondylitis	Inflammation of the intervertebral disk and adjacent vertebral bodies.
Encephalitis	Inflammation of the brain.
Encephalo-	Brain.
Granulomatous	Macrophage inflammation.
Hypomyelination	Defective formation of myelin in the spinal cord and brain.
Kyphosis	Dorsal deviation of the spinal column.
Leuko-	White matter of the CNS.
Malacia	Necrosis of the nervous tissue ("softening").
Meningitis	Inflammation of the meninges.
Myelo-	Spinal cord (or bone marrow).
Myositis	Inflammation of the skeletal muscles.
Myelitis	Inflammation of the spinal cord.
Non-suppurative	Lymphocytic and plasmacytic inflammation.
Osteomyelitis	Inflammation of the bone tissue and bone marrow.
Osteophyte	Pathological prolongation of a bone edge.
Polio-	Referring to the grey matter of the CNS.
Scoliosis	Lateral deviation of the spinal column.
Suppurative	Purulent (neutrophilic) inflammation.
Synovitis	Inflammation of the synovial membrane of a joint.

CNS: central nervous system (brain + spinal cord).

Suckling piglets

A diagnostic algorithm of the main nervous and locomotor disorders in suckling pigs based on clinical signs, lesions and laboratory techniques is presented in figure 1.

Congenital tremor is observed in newborn piglets usually delivered by gilts. It is classified in function of the presence (type A) or absence (type B) of histopathological lesions. If lesions are observed (hypomyelination, type A), a viral infection (classical swine fever virus) may be ruled out by different identification methods (PCR, IHC, ISH, isolation). Inherited autosomal recessive and sex-linked traits associated with Landrace and British Saddleback breeds should be investigated through genetic profiling and a historical assessment of the use of organophosphate insecticides in sows during gestation should be done.

Splay leg usually affects a small number of pigs in a litter. Although the clinical presentation is rather typical, histopathological confirmation can be achieved by special staining of frozen samples from the adductor muscles of 4 to 5-day old piglets. The percentage of animals affected by splay leg is sometimes much higher and can be related to infectious diseases affecting late gestation and causing delivery of weak-born piglets. An appropriate reproductive disease diagnostic procedure must be implemented in those cases (chapter 8).

Meningitis is discussed in the section the differential diagnosis in "growing and finishing pigs".

Encephalitis is usually caused by viral infections, being pseudorabies (Aujeszky's disease) the most common disease at this age. In pseudorabies, suckling and weaned pigs usually show nervous signs, while respiratory signs affect finishing and adult pigs. Reproductive failure (abortion) is also a common clinical sign in sows (chapter 8). The

pathological diagnosis is usually based on the histopathological examination, where microscopic lesions are indicative of non-suppurative encephalomyelitis, while the agent can be detected by means of specific laboratory techniques such as PCR, viral isolation or IHC.

Hypoglycemia can be caused by several factors affecting the sow such as poor nutrition, the presence of a disease, agalaxia, a cold or chilly environment and/or any disease in the piglet that impairs suckling. The diagnosis can be confirmed by blood biochemical profiles (reference range: 82.9 + 11.9 mg/dl) but predisposing factors should be identified. (Note: haematology and biochemistry reference ranges for pigs may vary with the age and breed, comparison between affected and non-affected piglets is therefore recommended).

Hypoxia may be due to dystocic/prolonged farrowing and torsion/rupture or PRRSV-induced lesions of the umbilical cord. Heated rooms with elevated levels of carbon monoxide have also been associated with hypoxia. Diagnosis is usually done by clinical signs and by exclusion.

Growing and finishing pigs

Nervous disorders

A diagnostic algorithm of the main nervous disorders in growing and finishing pigs based on clinical signs, lesions and laboratory techniques is shown in figure 2.

Enterotoxemic colibacillosis (oedema disease) is a disorder of healthy, rapidly growing pigs being fed a high-energy ration. Grossly, oedema is widespread, being especially obvious in the subcutis (palpebral/naso-facial) and viscera. Some pigs die within 24 hours. The results of the histopathological examination show bilateral polioencephalomalacia of the brain stem. Gross and

FIGURE 1. Main differential diagnoses in suckling pigs suffering from nervous and locomotor disorders.

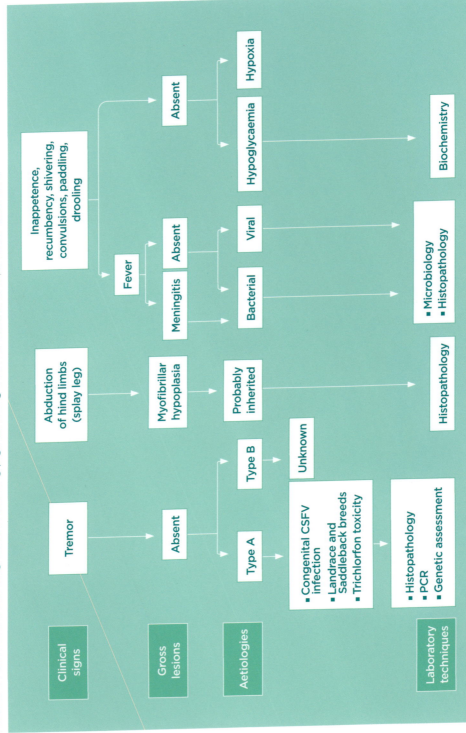

CSFV: classical swine fever virus.

FIGURE 2. Main differential diagnoses in growing-finishing pigs suffering from nervous disorders.

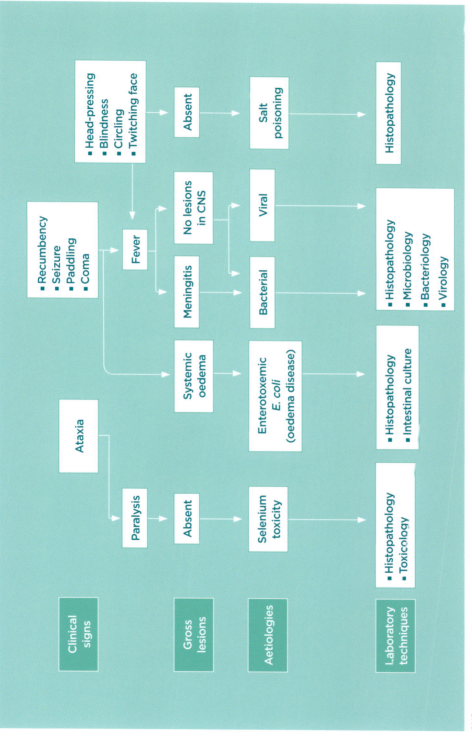

CNS: central nervous system.

microscopic lesions together with the isolation of β-hemolytic *Escherichia coli* are diagnostic of the disease.

Meningitis is a common consequence of septicaemia in neonatal and growing to finishing pigs, and is grossly observed (when evident) as an opacity of the leptomeninges. In pigs it is caused by several bacteria (*E. coli, Haemophilus parasuis, Streptococcus suis* or *Salmonella cholerae-suis*) that tend to cause fibrino-purulent inflammation of the leptomeninges, other viscera and joints. The identification of the causative agent by bacteriological culture or PCR from brain tissue, cerebrospinal fluid or meningeal swabs usually confirms the diagnosis.

Viral infections (Aujeszky's disease, rabies, classical swine fever, encephalomyocarditis, Teschen-Talfan, etc.) can be a serious problem in areas where these viruses are endemic. Some of them (Aujeszky's disease or classical swine fever viruses) usually lead to other systemic clinical symptoms or lesions that are helpful for their diagnosis. In the CNS, microscopic lesions are usually indicative of non-suppurative encephalomyelitis. Specific techniques such as PCR, viral isolation or IHC are necessary to identify the aetiology.

Salt poisoning (sodium chloride toxicity) occurs following over-consumption of sodium chloride and/or due to a limited availability of drinking water, followed by a rapid rehydration of the animals. The animals may show other specific nervous symptoms such as head-pressing, blindness, circling or twitching of the face. Polioencephalomalacia of the cerebral cortex (cerebrocortical neuronal necrosis) is sometimes observed microscopically accompanied by eosinophilic meningoencephalitis.

Selenium toxicity is sometimes observed since the margin between the daily requirements and the toxic dose is very narrow. The affected pigs are alert, recumbent and, depending on the affected areas of the spinal cord, may show paraparesis/paraplegia that eventually progresses to tetraplegia with flaccid paralysis of the rear limbs. Bilateral poliomyelomalacia of the cervical and lumbar segments of the spinal cord is observed histopathologically. Cutaneous lesions (rough hair coats, partial alopecia and/or sloughing of hoofs) may also appear in chronic courses.

Other toxicities (metals, plants, chemicals, etc.) are uncommon in intensively reared pigs. The affected animals may show a variety of clinical signs such as tremor, fasciculation, paralysis or seizures. Some of these toxicities may cause specific lesions in other organs. Hence, a complete necropsy and sample collection for histopathological examination and toxicological analysis are recommended.

Locomotor disorders

Alterations of the musculoskeletal system may be confused with certain nervous disorders because some nervous signs such as ataxia or paralysis (e. g. selenium toxicity) can be observed in both nervous and locomotor disorders. However, musculoskeletal disorders usually lack the typical nervous signs (seizures, paddling, circling, coma) and are manifested by other clinical symptoms such as lameness, muscular weakness or atrophy, trembling while standing, abnormal gait, muscle or joint swelling, fasciculation or pain. Apart from the external examination, clinical-pathological findings such as creatine kinase (CK) levels measured *in vivo* can be used to assess the presence or severity of muscular damage. On the other hand, the gross pathological appearance of the skeletal muscles can sometimes correspond to non-specific changes or artefacts; for this reason, histopathological examination is crucial to assess the presence and type of muscular damage. Samples from several muscles should be taken for histopathological examination, namely,

FIGURE 3. Main differential diagnoses in growing-finishing pigs suffering from musculoskeletal disorders. Abbreviations for laboratory techniques are included in brackets.

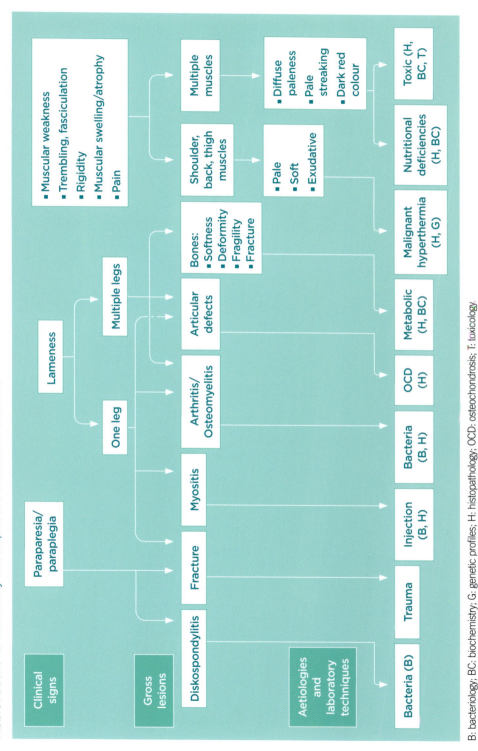

B: bacteriology; BC: biochemistry; G: genetic profiles; H: histopathology; OCD: osteochondrosis; T: toxicology.

from the shoulder, back and thigh muscles, the psoas and the diaphragm, since various myopathies affect different muscles. Figure 3 displays a diagnostic chart of the main loco-motor disorders in growing and finishing pigs based on clinical signs, lesions and laboratory techniques.

Diskospondylitis is usually due to septi-caemia and many bacteria can potentially be involved. The inflammation usually extends to the vertebral channel, compressing the spinal cord and causing hind limb paralysis (para-plegia). **Fractures** could be a consequence of trauma or electrocution at slaughter; vertebral fractures can also compress or damage the spinal cord causing paraplegia. Improperly formulated rations can lead to metabolic bone diseases increasing the risk of fractures (see next).

Focal **myositis** with purulent inflammation, necrosis or abscessation could be a conse-quence of injections or penetrating wounds, especially if these were contaminated.

Arthritis is usually caused by bacterial infections, and the type of exudate varies from purulent to fibrinous. Focal lesions are generally due to contaminated penetrating wounds, while multifocal arthritis is usually a consequence of septicaemia. Some of the most common forms of bacterial arthritis are caused by *H. parasuis* (Glasser's disease), *Arcanobacterium pyogenes*, *Mycoplasma hyosinoviae*, *Mycoplasma hyorhinis* and *Erysipelothrix rhusiopathiae* (erysipelas). In all these cases, bacteriological examination is the best option to confirm the presence of a bacterial infection. A histopathological exami-nation can be also performed to confirm or rule out other diagnoses (e. g. osteochondro-sis, trauma, neoplasia).

Osteochondrosis (OCD) is a hereditary disease that causes significant lameness in young breeding pigs and is characterised by focal or multifocal failure or endochondral ossification of the epiphysis and physis. It generally affects animals from 6 to 20 weeks of age, but it may extend to 18 months of age. It usually affects the shoulder, knee, elbow, carpal and intervertebral lumbar joints. Lesions are often bilateral and symmetrical. The articular cartilage surface may appear thickened, irregular, with very marked areas, the cartilage may be detached with expo-sure of the subchondral bone. Macroscopic inspection of articular cartilage may suggest OCD; however, longitudinal sections of the affected bones and a histopathological exam-ination are usually necessary for a correct evaluation and diagnostic confirmation.

Metabolic bone diseases in pigs are gen-erally of nutritional origin. **Rickets** affects growing pigs between 2-6 months age and **osteomalacia** is observed in adults. The pathogenesis for both involves a failure of bone mineralisation which is related to a deficiency of vitamin D or phosphorus in the diet. **Fibrous osteodystrophy** (FOD) is due to an inadequate proportion of calcium and phosphorus in the diet (Ca deficiency or P excess). Its physiopathology is associated with increased widespread bone resorption and replacement by fibrous tissue. The clini-cal signs and lesions of all these metabolic bone diseases are similar. Animals present with lameness, fractures and deformities (kyphosis, scoliosis). At necropsy, bones are easily bent and can usually be cut with a knife. In rickets, some animals may show prominent costochondral junctions ("rachitic rosary"), whereas in FOD some pigs may present with bilateral swelling of the max-illa or mandible. Diagnosis is usually based on clinical signs, lesions, histopathological examination and biochemical analysis of Ca, P and vitamin D levels in serum or diet.

Malignant hyperthermia (porcine stress syndrome) is an inherited autosomal reces-sive disease that occurs in homozygous pigs.

It is caused by a defect in cellular calcium channels (ryanodine receptor) that leads to excessive muscle contraction and heat production. The clinical disease appears during an episode of stress or halothane anaesthesia and consists of severe hyperthermia, muscle rigidity and rapid death. The shoulder, back and thigh muscles are most commonly affected. At necropsy, the affected muscles are pale, moist, swollen and appear "cooked". The clinical history together with the gross and histopathological lesions will suggest the diagnosis, which will be confirmed by genetic testing.

Nutritional myopathy is caused by a vitamin E and selenium (Se) deficiency and can also be manifested by hepatic (hepatosis dietetica) or cardiovascular (mulberry heart disease) alterations. It can be caused by unbalanced diets or diets containing compounds that destroy vitamin E or make it less available (diets high in polyunsaturated fatty acids or copper, mycotoxins, etc.). The postural muscles (medial muscles of limbs, neck, psoas), diaphragm, intercostal muscles, tongue and heart are the most commonly affected muscles. **Toxic myopathies** can be caused by the ingestion of high doses of ionophores (e. g. monensin), or less commonly, of toxic compounds derived from plants (gossypol present in cotton seed, *Cassia occidentalis*, etc). Their gross appearance can be non-specific and similar to nutritional or toxic myopathies, with paleness of the skeletal muscles or presence of chalky white streaks on the heart surface. Biochemical parameters such as CK levels may be markedly increased. A histopathological examination is necessary for the diagnosis, although diagnostic confirmation can be obtained by measuring the amount of vitamin E and Se in the diet, serum and liver, or by detecting/quantifying the toxic compounds in feed, stomach contents or liver.

Sows and boars

Nervous disorders in adult pigs are less frequent than in young pigs. However, in some naïve populations, several bacterial or viral infections can affect sows or boars. Toxic neuropathies such as selenium toxicity or salt poisoning can also affect adult animals. The clinical signs, lesions and diagnostic procedures are similar to those described in growing and finishing pigs.

Regarding locomotor disorders, lesions such as diskospondylitis, fractures, myositis, arthritis, FOD and nutritional or toxic myopathies can be observed in adults. Moreover, rickets and OCD, which are observed in growing pigs, can be seen in adults until closure of the growth plates. The time of closure depends on the individual and varies from 1 to 3.5 years. Infectious processes such as septicaemic arthritis are less common than in young pigs. Nevertheless, the incidence of **degenerative joint disease** (osteoarthrosis) increases with age. In these cases, the animals suffer from lameness; fibrillation or ulceration of the articular cartilage, osteophyte production and a thickening of the synovial membrane can be observed at necropsy. This condition can be monoarticular or polyarticular and its origin is multifactorial, its cause being a variety of diseases that have a common end stage (senility, osteochondrosis, infectious or traumatic arthritis, etc.). A histopathological examination or bacteriological analysis can be useful to identify any previous or predisposing diseases.

Otitis (inner or media) is generally due to progressive external otitis that can affect some cranial nerves and causes a vestibular syndrome, in which head-tilt is particularly common. In these cases, it is highly recommended to examine the tympanic bullae during the necropsy in order to look for exudates. Most cases are caused by bacterial infections; swabs can therefore be taken for microbiological analyses.

CLINICAL CASE

Clinical history

Fattening farm with 2000 pigs. The animals were moved to this farm at the age of 10 weeks and all the buildings were filled at 1-week intervals. During the first week after arrival, 70-80% of animals presented with diarrhoea and a small proportion of the pigs showed neuromuscular signs characterised by prostration and paraparesis. An infectious process (oedema disease) was suspected and the animals were treated with antibiotics and feed restriction. The clinical problem seemed to improve but when food was available to the pigs again, a significant increase of the number of animals with neurological signs was observed. A feeding problem was thus suspected. Skin reddening and alopecia were also observed in 30% of pigs. Morbidity and mortality finally affected 17.5% and 12% of animals, respectively.

Pathological analysis

Three live, 3-month-old male pigs (of 20 kg approx.) showing prostration with hyper-reactivity when handled, were submitted for necropsy. All of them had paresis with an abnormal position and typical "dog sitting posture". The animals presented with generalised and moderate alopecia (fig. 4) and multiple foci of cutaneous necrosis. Moreover, a ring-shaped area of skin necrosis around the coronary bands (fig. 5) was also observed.

The histopathological lesions consisted of symmetrical, bilateral, focal and severe lesions of poliomyelomalacia in the ventral horn of the cervical and lumbar intumescences of the spinal cord.

Toxicology

The analysis of the feed only yielded alterations in the selenium (Se) levels. The affected animals had a value of 9.6 mg/kg (recommended levels < 0.3 mg/kg). The affected pigs had serum Se levels between 1.13-1.80 mg/l, and were compared to control pigs from a different farm, whose levels ranged between 0.17 and 0.20 mg/l. Therefore, the Se concentration in serum was 6-to-9.7-fold higher in the clinically affected pigs than in the control pigs.

Discussion

This is a typical case of selenium toxicosis in pigs with neurological signs of paraparesis/paraplegia and dermatological symptoms of alopecia and hoof necrosis. Initially, diarrhoea and neurological signs suggested a possible infectious aetiology, most likely enterotoxemic colibacillosis. However, the antibiotics and feed restriction were unsuccessful and the clinical symptoms worsened after the treatment. A pathological analysis revealed a necrotic (malacic) process in the spinal cord, which explained the hind limb paresis. The toxicological analysis of the feed and serum confirmed the diagnosis.

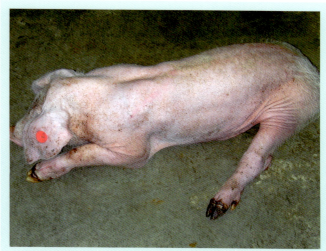

Figure 4. Pig clinically affected by selenium toxicosis. The animal is prostrated, with abnormal hind limb position and presents with moderate emaciation and generalised alopecia.

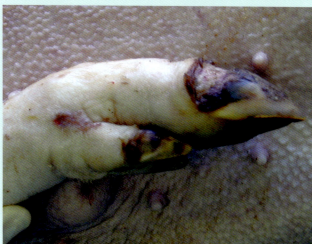

Figure 5. Pig clinically affected by selenium toxicosis. Distal third of a hind limb with severe erosive and necrotic coronary band of the hoof.

10

Laboratory diagnosis of cutaneous disorders

INTRODUCTION

The skin is the largest organ in the body and consists of the epidermis, dermis, subcutis and adnexa (hair follicles and sebaceous, sweat and other glands). Skin diseases may involve the skin only or be a cutaneous manifestation of an internal disease. Thus, skin diseases in the pig can be broadly divided into two groups: those conditions that only affect the skin and have minimal effect on the animal, and those that are the signs of a more generalised disease. It is therefore necessary to take an accurate clinical history, followed by a thorough clinical examination of the whole animal first and then of the skin.

CLINICAL AND PATHOLOGICAL EXAMINATION

The information should be obtained from an on-farm examination and it should be as complete as possible. An examination of the farm is useful to identify risk factors for some skin diseases. Poor hygiene, high environmental temperatures and outdoor housing may lead to the appearance of specific diseases such as bacterial pyodermas, traumatic lesions or sunburn/photosensitisation, respectively. Moreover, several factors should be kept in mind during the collection of the clinical history, such as the proportion of affected pigs, the age of the affected group, the presence of widespread disease, the onset of the problem (sudden or present for some time), and response to treatment.

With all these data, the veterinary surgeon may have a serious suspicion of the condition that is affecting the animals. However, a clinical examination with special emphasis on the distribution and morphology of the skin lesions is crucial to obtain an accurate diagnosis. In some cases, it is necessary to take skin biopsies for histopathology during surgical procedures, necropsies or slaughter inspection to reach a definitive diagnosis. In these cases, it is very important to submit a well-detailed macroscopic description of the lesions using the correct terminology for skin lesions (table 1).

DIFFERENTIAL DIAGNOSES

Classifying skin disorders by age is somehow difficult since many conditions affect different age ranges. However, this section tries to describe the most usual skin problems and to include them in the most commonly affected age groups. Finally, those conditions that affect a broad age group are specifically mentioned.

Suckling and growing piglets

Several infectious and non-infectious conditions may affect piglets during the suckling and growing period. However, only some of the most common conditions will be mentioned.

Exudative epidermitis (greasy pig disease) is caused by *Staphylococcus hyicus* and is one of the most common skin disorders in pigs. The morbidity rate can be high but the mortality rate is low. The affected piglets show brownish exudates around the eyes, pinnae, snout, chin and medial area of the legs; in severe cases they spread to the ventral thorax and abdomen, giving the animal an overall "greasy" appearance. Grossly, the epidermis is thickened, scabby, with scaling. Diagnosis is usually made by histopathological examination and bacterial culture of a regional lymph node.

Skin necrosis is usually observed in suckling piglets and affects the knees, hocks, toes, elbows, teats, coronary bands and soles of the feet. The lesions are due to trauma from hard abrasive floors.

TABLE 1. Definition and examples of some specific terms used to describe skin lesions macroscopically.

Term	Definition	Examples
Crust	Dried exudate on the skin surface.	Exudative epidermitis, swine pox.
Erosion	Superficial loss of skin (part of the epidermis).	Vesicle rupture or surface trauma.
Lichenification	Rough, thickened epidermis secondary to persistent rubbing, scratching, or irritation.	Mange.
Macule	Flat, circumscribed area (< 1 cm) where the skin colour has changed.	Erysipelas, porcine dermatitis and nephropathy syndrome.
Nodule	Raised, firm, circumscribed lesion (> 1 cm in diameter).	Neoplasm, granuloma.
Papule	Raised, firm, circumscribed area (< 1 cm in diameter).	Insect bite.
Pustule	Raised superficial accumulation of purulent fluid within the epidermis.	Bacterial infection.
Scales	Flaky skin, dry or oily.	Ectoparasites, exudative epidermitis.
Ulcer	Deep loss of skin (loss of epidermis and exposure of dermis).	Flank, ear or tail-biting.
Vesicles	Raised, circumscribed, fluid-filled lesion (< 1 cm in diameter).	Viral infections (e. g. foot-and-mouth disease).
Wheal	Small oedematous area of the skin, usually itchy.	Insect bite.

Ear necrosis may have a uni or bilateral distribution and can affect the tip, the base or be so severe that most of the ear is lost. It is related with traumatic lesions (biting or self-inflicted trauma) contaminated by secondary bacteria. It can also be secondary to chronic vascular disorders causing cyanosis of the ears. Gross examination will generally suggest a diagnosis.

Finishing pigs

Erysipelas is caused by an infection by *Erysipelothrix rhusiopathiae*. The systemic infection is the result of a sepsis causing different lesions such as endocarditis, arthritis or cutaneous lesions. The skin lesions consist of square to rhomboidal, pink to dark purple macules or papules. Erythematous lesions that do not necessarily correspond with erysipelas are sometimes observed in systemic infections. The detection of *E. rhusiopathiae* in several tissues (heart, lungs, liver, spleen, kidney, joints, skin), by microbiological culture or PCR, will confirm the diagnosis.

Porcine dermatitis and nephropathy syndrome (PDNS) is suspected to be an immune-related systemic disorder (immunocomplex disease) affecting the skin and kidneys. Its aetiology is unknown but it has been strongly related to porcine circovirus type 2 infections; however, a definitive proof of causality is still lacking. Cutaneous lesions are accompanied by rapid weight loss and depression. Lesions vary from multifocal areas of erythema, macules or papules to brown or black crusts starting on the hindquarters and extending to the ears, face, lower limbs and scrotum or vulva. Macroscopic skin lesions and renal lesions (petechiae) are rather suggestive of this condition. However, a definitive diagnosis is generally reached by histopathological examination, with the observation of necrotising vasculitis.

Conditions affecting all age groups

Dermatophytosis

Dermatophytosis (ringworm) affects different age groups and usually appears in buildings with poor sanitation. The lesions appear as well-demarcated, round alopecic areas of different sizes, sometimes with scales or crust formation. The diagnosis can be confirmed by collection of hairs from the periphery of the lesions and subsequent microscopic examination or fungal culture. It seldom occurs in pigs.

Sarcoptic mange

Sarcoptic mange is a common dermatosis in pigs with a worldwide distribution caused by the burrowing mite *Sarcoptes scabiei*. It is highly contagious and spreads by close physical contact. In the early stages, infestation may not be apparent. The clinical signs are marked pruritus, erythema, papules, crusts, excoriation and lichenification, particularly on the ears, flanks, abdomen and rump. The cutaneous response reflects inflammation produced by keratinocyte damage and the development of cutaneous hypersensitivity (type I) to the mite antigens.

Two typical forms of dermatitis are commonly observed in *S. scabiei* infected pigs. The hypersensitive form occurs following primary infestations and is typically seen in fattening pigs. The hyperkeratotic form causes crusted lesions in a small number of adults. These lesions tend to be localised, especially in the ear pinnae, and often contain large mite populations.

The diagnosis is based on the history, clinical examination and identification of mites. Different diagnostic tests can be performed to determine the prevalence of sarcoptic mange: identification of mites in ear scrapings, dermatitis score, scratching index and detection of specific serum antibodies.

The scrapings can be examined under a stereo microscope to detect the presence of *S.scabiei* after exposure at 28 ºC for 30 min. It is recommended to perform an indirect examination of the scrapings using digestion of the crusts with 10% potassium hydroxide followed by a sedimentation-flotation technique with sucrose.

Insect bites

- **Lice.** Pigs may be infested by the sucking louse *Haematopinus suis* (hog louse), which lives around the ears, axillae and groin. The clinical signs associated with lice infestation are pruritus, scales, crusts and excoriation. Severe infestation with this type of lice can produce anaemia. The hog louse plays a role in the transmission of some infectious agents such as swine pox virus or *Mycoplasma suis*. Diagnosis is made on the basis of clinical signs and by identification of lice on the skin.
- **Flies, mosquitoes and black flies.** Blood-feeding dipterans cause discomfort, dermatitis, and anaemia when they are present in large amounts, especially in young pigs. Fly bites may produce painful papules and wheals with variable pruritus. Diagnosis is based on the history and clinical signs.

CLINICAL CASE

Clinical history

During the slaughtering of a batch of pigs, some of the carcasses showed widespread reddening of the skin due to the presence of erythematous papular dermatitis (fig. 1). Some other individuals also had this type of lesion, although at a lesser degree and more dispersed. The vets considered a type of allergic reaction to be the most likely cause and therefore decided to record it in the inspection report. It was necessary to investigate the problem on the farm of origin and assess the situation by age, feed quality, environmental conditions and health programmes.

Differential diagnosis

Exudative epidermitis (greasy pig disease), nutritionally induced dermatoses, vesicular and viral dermatoses, hyperkeratinisation, insect bites, ringworm or pityriasis rosea.

Farm investigation

Piglets and sows did not show these types of lesions previously. In some growing pigs and finishers, hypersensitivity reactions were evident, but their aspect was less clear than in carcasses after scalding. The results of the skin scrapings from papular lesions on the neck, shoulders and back were negative in the 15 analysed pigs. The analysis of the feed indicated that the concentrations of feed supplement and mycotoxins were within the normal range; the environmental conditions were correct too. Apparently, there had been no changes in the medication, vaccination and deworming schedules, with the exception of the recent substitution of ivermectin by doramectin.

Although no cases of mange had been recorded on the farm since the introduction of ivermectin a few years earlier, the vets decided to carry out an assessment of the state of this disease. They calculated the scratching index (SI) for growing and finishing animals on the farm (SI = 0.5). Moreover, the average dermatitis score (ADS) was determined at slaughter by assessment of the extent of the lesions in a sample batch. The results for the 75 pigs

were: Grade 0 = 36, Grade 1 = 34, Grade 2 = 4 and Grade 3 = 1 (ADS = 0.6).

At slaughter, samples of skin were scraped from the ears of 75 fattening pigs with a curette. The scrapings were observed directly for the presence of mites under a binocular microscope; 8 out of 75 pigs were positive. The negative scrapings were subjected to indirect examination using digestion of the crusts with 10% potassium hydroxide (KOH) followed by a flotation technique with sucrose; with this technique 4 out of 67 animals were also

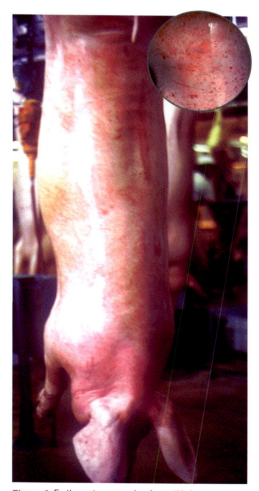

Figure 1. Erythematous papular dermatitis in a slaughtered pig (grade 2-3).

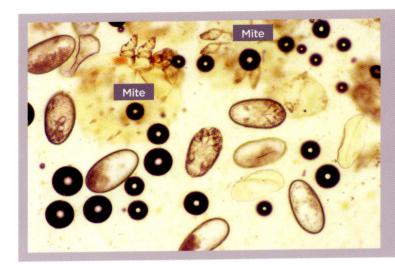

Figure 2. Positive scraping (*S. scabiei* mites) using digestion with KOH 10%, followed by flotation technique with sucrose.

positive (fig. 2). Hence, a total of 12 fattening pigs were positive for *S. scabiei*.

Serological tests were not performed due to the unavailability of this technique.

Discussion

Pruritus is a common symptom of sarcoptic mange, and measuring rubbing behaviour by using the SI can be useful in growing and finishing animals. The threshold value commonly used for SI is 0.4; some reports indicated a significant correlation between ADS > 0.5 and the presence of the mite on a farm. However, these reports also showed that only 45% of the animals with generalised dermatitis were positive for *S. scabiei*; therefore, this method is not considered a reliable tool on an individual basis.

Microscopic examination of ear scrapings is a very specific method for sarcoptic mange. In this clinical case, the positive results obtained by this method confirmed the presence of *S. scabiei* and the disease (hypersensitive sarcoptic mange) on the farm. Nevertheless, this method has a low sensitivity and the real prevalence of the disease on the farm was underestimated.

The standard control protocol with two treatments with ivermectin usually gives successful results. However, some failures have been observed after the one-shot-injection with doramectin.

A summary of the methods commonly used in swine sarcoptic mange is shown in table 2.

TABLE 2. Advantages and disadvantages of diagnostic methods used in swine sarcoptic mange.

	Scratching index (SI)	Average dermatitis score (ADS)	Ear scratching	Serology
Advantages	▪ Simple and economic. ▪ Decreases after treatment.	▪ Easy, fast and economic. ▪ Specific for grades 2 and 3.	▪ Definitive if positive results. ▪ High specificity.	▪ High sensitivity in finishers. ▪ Appropriate for eradication programmes.
Disadvantages	▪ Not useful for early diagnosis. ▪ Subjective. ▪ Low specificity. ▪ Negative results in parasitised piglets and positive results in non-parasitised sows can sometimes be observed.	▪ Not useful for early diagnosis. ▪ Long delays between treatment and dermatitis improvement.	▪ Low sensitivity (negative results do not rule out the presence of mange).	▪ Elevated costs. ▪ Low availability. ▪ Not adequate for sows. ▪ Long delays between treatment and decrease of antibodies.

11

Conclusions

The present guide intends to offer general principles of laboratory diagnostic orientation. It combines key information on clinical and pathological findings with important concepts about the laboratory techniques used by swine vets in their daily practice. As end-users of laboratory results, practitioners are expected know how to take samples and submit them, what type of test will provide them the necessary information and, finally, how to interpret the result obtained.

As mentioned previously, laboratories are able to assist vets by providing analytical results. However, the final diagnosis of a disease or poor performance problem or the decision to control or eradicate a disease must be made by the submitting veterinary surgeon. In the end, the practitioner is the only person able to assess the importance of the laboratory results in relation to other factors implicated in the abovementioned scenarios.

It is worth highlighting that the veterinary surgeon has a significant impact on the reliability of the analytical result and should therefore try to maximise the benefits offered by laboratory testing. This can be done by:

- Defining a clear goal for the submission: what is the question to be answered?
- Working with laboratories that can reliably offer analyses subject to appropriate quality assurance.
- Selecting the appropriate samples from representative pigs or population of animals, and submitting them correctly.
- Being aware of the strengths and limitations of laboratory analyses, and interpreting their results accordingly.

In case the analytical results do not meet the vet's expectations, it is important to discuss this issue with the personnel from the laboratory. Moreover, practitioners must also be open to modifying their clinical diagnostic hypotheses and/or reinterpreting the pathological findings observed.

REFERENCES

1. CALLÉN A, HERNÁNDEZ E. *La sarna porcina: diagnóstico, control y erradicación.* Cuadernos de Campo Ivomec, 2003.
2. CASTRO A. E., HEUSCHELE W. P. *Veterinary Diagnostic Virology.* Section I: Viral diagnosis: General considerations. Mosby Year Book, 1992.
3. EpiCentre Website: http://epicentre.massey.ac.nz/
4. FreeCalc: http://www.ausvet.com.au/content.php?page=software#freecalc
5. LELAND D. S. *Clinical Virology.* WB Saunders Company, 1996.
6. MUIRHEAD M. R., ALEXANDER T. J. L. *Managing pig health and the treatment of disease,* 5M enterprises, 1997.
7. MORILLA A., YOON K. J., ZIMMERMAN J. J. *Trends in emerging viral infections of swine.* Iowa State Press, 2002.
8. PFEIFFER D. (2002). *Veterinary Epidemiology:* An Introduction: http://www2.vetmed.wisc.edu/education/courses/epi/Pfeiffer.pdf
9. RADOSTITS O. M., GAY C.C., HINCHCLIFF K.W., CONSTABLE P. D. *Veterinary Medicine:* A textbook of the diseases of cattle, horses, sheep, pigs and goats. 10th ed. Saunders, 2007.
10. SEGALÉS J., DOMINGO M. *La necropsia en el Ganado porcino, diagnóstico anatomopatológico y toma de muestras.* Boehringer Ingelheim, 2003.
11. SEGALÉS J., RAMOS-VARA J. A., DURAN C. O., *et al.* Diagnosing infectious diseases using *in situ* hybridization. Swine Health and Production, 1999, 7:125-128.
12. SIMS L. D., GLASTONBURY J. R. W. Pathology of the pig - A diagnostic guide. Pig Research and Development Corporation and Agriculture, Victoria, Australia, 1996.
13. SMETS K, VERCRUYSSE J. Evaluation of different methods for the diagnosis of scabies in swine. Veterinary Parasitology, 2000, 90:137-145.
14. STRAW B. E., D'ALLAIRE S., MENGELING W. L., TAYLOR D. J. *Diseases of swine.* 8th edition. Iowa State University Press, 1999.
15. STRAW B. E., D'ALLAIRE S., MENGELING W. L., TAYLOR D. J. *Diseases of swine.* 9th edition. Blackwell Publishing, 2006.
16. The Indiana Animal Disease Diagnostic Laboratory at Purdue University West Lafayette, IN: https://www.addl.purdue.edu/SampleSubmission/Users_Guide.pdf
17. The Iowa State University webpage. Veterinary Diagnostic and Production Animal Medicine: http://vetmed.iastate.edu/diagnostic-lab/user-guide
18. THRUSFIELD, M. *Veterinary Epidemiology.* 3rd edition. Wiley-Blackwell, 2007.
19. WALL R., SHEARER D. Veterinary Entomology. Chapman & Hall.
20. Winepi (Working in Epidemiology): http://www.winepi.net/, 1997.
21. Win Episcope 2.0: http://www.clive.ed.ac.uk/cliveCatalogueItem.asp?id=B6BC9009-C10F-4393-A22D-48F436516AC4
22. Wong's Virology webpage: http://virology-online.com/
23. YTREHUS B., CARLSON C. S., EKMAN S. Etiology and pathogenesis of osteochondrosis. Veterinary Pathology, 2007, 44:429-448.
24. ZACHARY J., McGAVIN M.D. *Pathological basis of veterinary disease.* Mosby-Elsevier, 2012.
25. ZIMMERMAN J. J., KARRIKER L. A., RAMÍREZ A., SCHWARTZ K. J., STEVENSON G. W. *Diseases of swine.* 10th edition. John Wiley & Sons, Inc, 2012.

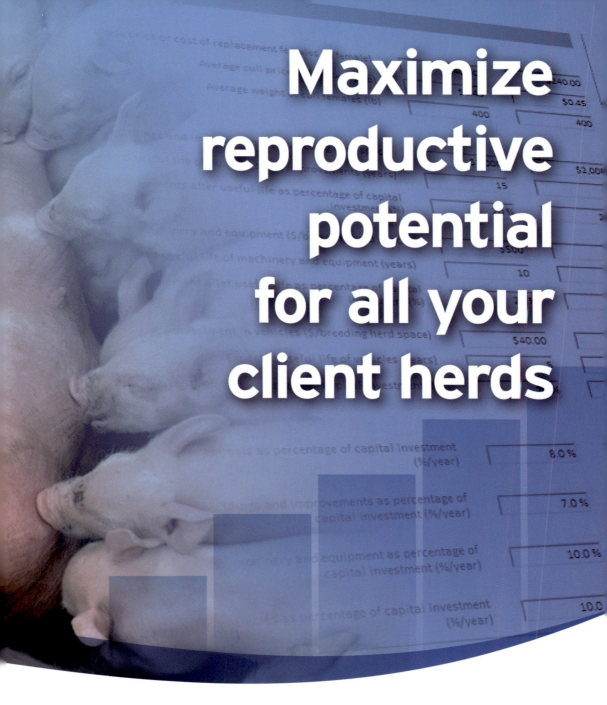

Maximize reproductive potential for all your client herds

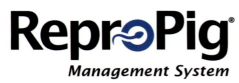

Repr⊙Pig®

Management System

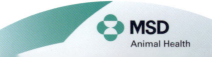

MSD Animal Health

ReproPig® Management System provides tools for breeding herd success

Helping your clients succeed is your job. Helping you succeed is ours. That's why MSD Animal Health created the ReproPig® Management System. It's a web-based platform accessible 24/7 and is designed to identify areas of improvement within the breeding herd. The goal is to help you and your clients achieve optimal reproductive performance – and offer customized, specific solutions for each farm.

A ReproPig review:

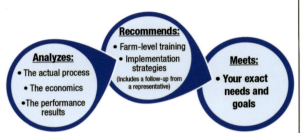

Analyzes:
- The actual process
- The economics
- The performance results

Recommends:
- Farm-level training
- Implementation strategies

(Includes a follow-up from a representative)

Meets:
- **Your exact needs and goals**

The web-based platform consists of four different areas to evaluate the best approach to reproductive efficiency. **The Audit** presents an objective view of the operation. **The Economic Data Review** calculates the return on investment (ROI) of recommended changes. **The Training** section includes customized video presentations from industry experts to help meet goals. **The Products** section determines which products will help maximize reproductive productivity.

Potential ReproPig benefits:

- Improve uniformity and batch management
- Maximize AI logistics, including delivery and scheduling
- Reduce NPDs to achieve more pigs/sow/year
- Manage workforce and facilities more efficiently
- Maximize the reproductive life cycle for more profitability
- Increase sow longevity by minimizing culling and replacement rates
- Reduce boar semen costs with a single fixed-time insemination

ReproPig helps you maximize productivity and efficiency.

Contact your MSD Animal Health representative today to review the web-based ReproPig Management System.

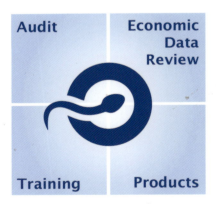

Audit

Economic Data Review

Training

Products

ReproPig® Web Platform

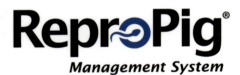

RebroPig®

Management System

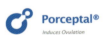
Porceptal®
Induces Ovulation

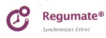
Regumate®
Synchronizes Estrus

PG 600®
Induces Estrus

Planate®
Induces Farrowing

GL/RPR/0114/0001

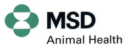
MSD
Animal Health